FITNESS
A Lifetime
Commitment

SECOND EDITION

David K. Miller
T. Earl Allen

**University of North Carolina
at Wilmington**

Burgess Publishing Company
Minneapolis, Minnesota

Editorial: Wayne Schotanus, Elisabeth Sövik, Anne Heller
Copy editor: Robert Bergad
Production: Morris Lundin, Pat Barnes, Melinda Berndt
Composition: K.F. Merrill Company
Cover design: Cheri Wyman, Wyman Graphics

Burgess Publishing Company
7108 Ohms Lane
Minneapolis, Minnesota 55435

J I H G F E

To our wives, Roselyn and Johanna

CONTENTS

PREFACE

This book is designed primarily for college men and women enrolled in courses in physical fitness, body conditioning, or foundations of physical activity. The objectives are to provide a clear understanding of the purpose of physical exercise, to enable the student to evaluate his or her own level of physical fitness, and to design a personalized exercise program that can be beneficial throughout life.

Throughout this book, the word *exercise* and the term *exercise program* will be used. Unless otherwise stated, both are interpreted to mean an organized, regular program of physical activity designed to develop or maintain the components of physical fitness.

Some authors define *physical fitness* as the capacity for sustained physical activity without excessive fatigue or as the capacity to perform everyday activities with reserve energy for emergency situations. Many persons may incorrectly classify themselves as physically fit by these definitions, and it is especially incorrect to accept these definitions when the relations between inactivity and health are considered. For the purposes of this book, no definition of physical fitness will be given. However, the concept will be taken to include circulorespiratory endurance, muscular strength and endurance, flexibility, and weight management.

This second edition has been revised and expanded to fulfill the desired objectives better. Recent research and information concerning heart disease, strength training, exercise-induced injuries, the female response to training, nutrition, and depression have been included. Furthermore, additional emphasis has been given to the development of an individualized exercise prescription.

As in the previous edition, key terms, the pages on which they are found, and behavioral objectives are listed at the beginning of each chapter. Fulfillment of the objectives will accomplish the purposes of the book. The key terms appear in boldface roman type, and other words that the authors wish to emphasize are italicized.

Each chapter is designed to stand alone, and the sequence of chapters may be rearranged to meet the needs of a particular group of students. To develop a clear understanding of heart disease, exercise prescription, and training responses to exercise, the student should possess a basic knowledge of the anatomy and physiology of the circulatory, respiratory, and muscular systems. Chapters 8, 9, and 10 include this information for the student whose background is inadequate. However, important concepts other than those of basic anatomy and physiology are also included in those chapters.

The appendix includes a test for self-evaluation of circulo-respiratory endurance, a table for physical fitness classification, and percentile scores for Cooper's Twelve-Minute Run. The glossary clarifies terms not fully defined in the text.

The sixteen accompanying laboratory sessions provide another avenue for meeting the behavioral objectives. These self-evaluating sessions also give the instructor and student an opportunity to assess the student's needs for an individualized physical fitness program.

The authors wish to express their appreciation to the many students and colleagues who directly and indirectly contributed to the writing of both editions of this book and to the publishers who have graciously allowed the reproduction of tables. Most grateful acknowledgment is also extended to Sharon Brewington for her assistance in the preparation of the manuscript, to Talmsi Schultz and Jan Allen for the illustrations, and to Daniel Noel and Dillon Bryant for the photography. David Cameron, T. L. Doolittle, A. W. Faris, Ed Hooks, Marylou Morgan, and Doug Smith are thanked for their early reviews of the manuscript. A special debt is owed to Bob Clayton for assistance and encouragement throughout the project.

KEY TERMS
Body image (p. 2)
Hypokinetic disease (p. 3)
Neuromuscular efficiency (p. 4)
Self-concept (p. 2)
Self-estimate (p. 2)
Self-image (p. 2)

BEHAVIORAL OBJECTIVES
Upon completion of this chapter, the student should be able to:
1. Define the key terms listed above.
2. Describe five major changes and problems that the human population has experienced in modern times.
3. List and discuss at least six benefits to be gained from a regular exercise program.

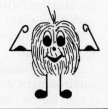

People are designed for physical activity. Primitive humans had to be able to run, climb, jump, and throw to provide for their needs and to escape constant threats to their lives. They had to be physically fit: only the fittest survived. This capacity for physical activity remains present in modern people. Even the developing embryo moves within the uterus long before the mother becomes aware of it. After the infant is born, the parents can hardly wait for the child to crawl and walk, but encouragement to move is not really needed: the desire to walk, skip, run, and play is present from the start. Often during adolescence and adulthood, however, habits of inactivity are developed and permitted to become a part of daily living.

The development of these habits of inactivity is primarily due to the presence of labor-saving devices. One hundred years ago, only 6% of the energy used to produce goods was mechanical; the remaining 94% was generated by human or animal muscle power. Today, however, as much as 96% of all energy used is mechanical, and 70% of the working population performs nonphysical tasks. Power steering and power brakes, driven lawn mowers, remote-control television, and similar devices have made the American people weaker and lazier. Associated with this life-style have been increases in the number of people experiencing degenerative and cardiovascular diseases, excessive weight gain, lower back pain, and mental illness. Also, the **self-concept, self-image, body image,** and **self-estimate** of many individuals have suffered owing to lack of movement and physical deterioration.

In addition, people today have experienced more changes and crises than any other generation. The knowledge explosion and the use of computers, the population explosion, increased leisure time, the energy crisis, pollution, and the frenzied pace of living are but a few of the major changes and problems facing the world today. These changes and crises have altered the human environment much too fast. Mental strain and stress have resulted, creating a way of life that is biologically and psychologically unsuitable. To compensate for the daily pressures that they must face, people depend on coffee to awaken them in the morning, alcohol and tranquilizers to calm their disturbed nerves, and sleeping pills to help them rest at night. However, these drinks and pills have not succeeded in providing the desired results: mental illness is more prevalent now than ever before.

Even though these habits of inactivity have developed and our environment has changed, the very important and basic human need for movement has remained. Movement is refreshing: the simple act of opening and closing the hand or tapping the foot can be a relief to someone who must remain sitting or standing for a long period of time. The morning and afternoon breaks from one's work are often refreshing due to the moving or walking associated with them. Movement is necessary even during sleep to promote circulation.

Movement is also related to one's self-concept. Self-image, body image, and self-estimate constitute self-concept; an individual who ranks low on any one of them will probably have a poor self-concept. A successful exercise program can improve one's self-image and self-estimate. It can make a person feel good and develop a positive view of life. Also, movement and action are essential for the development of one's body image.

An individual who has a healthy body image, self-image, and self-estimate is more likely to attempt new physical activities, and participation in these can provide opportunities for social recognition and development of friendships. Various group activities can also develop one's ability to work harmoniously with others and to adjust to their wishes and feelings. Often a togetherness of the group emerges and carries over into situations other than those found in sports. Many persons fail to enjoy the social interaction that can be experienced in a program of physical activity owing to their unwarranted concern about physical appearance and performance and their low estimate of potential success. A specified level of physical fitness, which in turn may improve one's self-concept, should be developed prior to participation in leisure activities if maximum social benefits are to be gained from this participation.

Perhaps an even more important aspect of movement is the possible prevention of degenerative and cardiovascular diseases. The law of use and disuse dictates that one must use one's body if it is to be developed and maintained at a high level of efficiency, and that, if one fails to do so, the body will deteriorate (**hypokinetic disease**). There is more and more evidence to indicate that a regular exercise program keeps the cardiovascular system, as well as other systems of the body, in good condition. Exercise develops the heart and lungs, so that they are able to supply oxygen to the muscles without strain. Regular exercise has been reported to improve coronary circulation and to reduce the risk of obstructive arterial disease. An exercise program helps one maintain desirable weight, and it also helps prevent the weight gain, lower back pain, loss of flexibility, and other degenerative diseases often associated with aging. Improvement in muscular strength and endurance, blood supply, innervation, and flexibility enhance **neuromuscular efficiency,** which increases the participant's chances for success in leisure activities.

In addition, emotional needs are related to the need for movement. The human body has identical reactions to mental and physical stress. This means that a physically fit person is better prepared to adapt to and cope with mental stress. Physical activity provides an outlet that enables a person to "let go," to release instinctive aggressive drives, and to relieve stifled anger and hostility. It also can be effective therapy for depression. Fulfilling the goals of an exercise program and experiencing the mental peace and physical relaxation that usually follow an exercise session enhance the participant's emotional health. Many Americans would be well advised to seek peace and relaxation this way rather than through alcohol or drugs.

From all the reasons given here, it should be apparent that a regular physical exercise program is not a luxury but a necessity. There are many types and variations of exercise programs, and each individual should select one according to personal interests and needs. However, everyone should know the why, as well as the how, of physical exercise. More people would follow a regular exercise regimen if they truly understood its purpose.

KEY TERMS

Angina pectoris (p. 9)
Atherosclerosis (p. 8)
Coronary heart disease (CHD) (p. 8)
Fibrous plaque (p. 10)
High-density lipoprotein (HDL) (p. 13)
Hypercholesterolemia (p. 12)
Hyperlipidemia (p. 12)
Hypertension (p. 12)
Ischemia (p. 9)
Low-density lipoprotein (LDL) (p. 13)
Myocardial infarction (p. 9)
Retrograde murmur (p. 16)
Rheumatic heart disease (p. 17)
Serum cholesterol (p. 12)
Serum triglyceride (p. 12)
Stenosis (p. 16)

BEHAVIORAL OBJECTIVES

Upon completion of this chapter, the student
should be able to:

1. Define the key terms listed above.
2. Identify three theories that seek to explain
   the origin and development of
   atherosclerosis.
3. Describe four steps in the progressive
   development of coronary heart disease.
4. Identify three primary and seven
   secondary risk factors associated with the
   development of coronary heart disease
   according to the multiple risk factor
   theory.
5. Identify safe ranges for blood pressure
   and desirable levels for serum cholesterol,
   serum triglyceride, and HDL cholesterol.
6. List six risk factors that are positively
   influenced by exercise.
7. List three characteristics of a highly
   trainable postinfarction patient that are
   somewhat controllable.

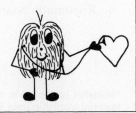

Cardiovascular (CV) diseases are the major cause of death in the United States today.* In 1977, 52% of all deaths were from diseases of the heart and blood vessels (CV disease), as shown in Figure 2-1. Of the deaths attributed to CV disease, 64.8% were due to heart attack and 18.5% were from stroke [1]. The remaining deaths were due to conditions such as rheumatic heart disease, hypertensive disease, and congenital heart disease. Difficult to accept at any age, death is an inescapable part of living. However, it is particularly tragic when it strikes prematurely those who are in the prime of life. Forty percent of the deaths in men ages 40 to 59 are attributable to a special type of CV disease called **coronary heart disease**.

More than 40 million Americans have some form of CV disease. Of this number about 34,400,000 have hypertension. Over 4,000,000 have CHD, and another 1,850,000 have rheumatic heart disease. Annually approximately 1,820,000 Americans experience stroke [1].

As can be seen in Figure 2-2, the economic cost of these disorders is staggering. It is estimated that the consequence of CV disease in 1980 was about $41 billion. The real tragedy is that much of the expense and human suffering might be avoidable.

In the past decade we have seen the deaths from CV disease decline slightly. Health care professionals are reluctant to conclude that a reduced occurrence is responsible. They prefer to explain the decreased mortality rate by citing improved medical diagnostic ability and disease management techniques as well as a general public that is more enlightened about heart disease.

Basic knowledge of causes, preventive measures, and modern treatments should enable one to respond intelligently to cardiovascular danger signs that might occur at some future date. Owing to the limited scope of this manual, only a few of the more common types of heart disorders are described, as follows:

1. Coronary heart disease (resulting in angina pectoris or myocardial infarction)
2. Congenital defects
3. Valvular lesions
4. Rhythm disorders
5. Rheumatic heart disease

*Statistics presented in connection with heart disease were taken from the latest material available from DHEW (1977) and the American Heart Association (1980).

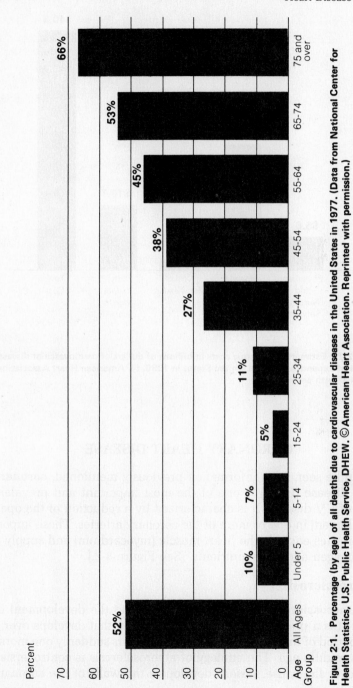

Figure 2-1. Percentage (by age) of all deaths due to cardiovascular diseases in the United States in 1977. (Data from National Center for Health Statistics, U.S. Public Health Service, DHEW. © American Heart Association. Reprinted with permission.)

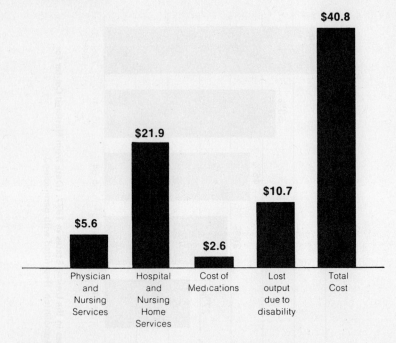

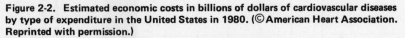

Figure 2-2. Estimated economic costs in billions of dollars of cardiovascular diseases by type of expenditure in the United States in 1980. (©American Heart Association. Reprinted with permission.)

CORONARY HEART DISEASE

As can be seen from information previously mentioned, **coronary heart disease** (CHD) is one of the most important and prevalent types of CV disease. It is characterized by a reduction of the open area (lumen) in one or more of the coronary arteries. These important arteries encircle the heart muscle (myocardium) and supply it with oxygen and other nutrients. (See Figure 8-2.)

Atherosclerosis

Atherosclerosis is a major contributor to the development of CHD. It is a progressive pathologic condition that develops over a long period of time, not something that appears suddenly one morning in middle age. The etiology of atherosclerosis is controversial. Whatever the cause, *lesions* develop in the walls of the coronary arteries. Over the years, this pathologic process continues until the blood flow is seriously reduced (a condition known as **ischemia**) or even until the vessel becomes completely occluded. The slowly developing atherosclerotic process finally becomes dramatically manifest in the occurrence of angina pectoris or myocardial infarction (heart attack).

Angina Pectoris

The term **angina pectoris** means chest pain. This disorder is caused by the inability of the coronary arteries to supply the myocardium (heart muscle) with adequate oxygen. The pain is usually not present when one is at rest but is precipitated by physical exertion. It is described as excruciating, often radiating from the sternum to the shoulders, jaw, and arms. It usually subsides with the cessation of the activity. Depending on the severity of the condition, treatment includes diet and drug therapy, exercise, or surgical procedures.

Myocardial Infarction

A **myocardial infarction** is a heart attack. The term *infarct* refers to an area of dead tissue resulting from inadequate circulation in the myocardium. If a coronary artery becomes occluded by a clot (thrombus) or by some other material, the tissue beyond that point is deprived of blood. The tissue dies (necrosis), and the area is permanently damaged. If the damaged area is large enough, the victim dies. A milder condition can be treated successfully, and many patients can be rehabilitated. As is the case with angina pectoris, drug therapy and exercise are important in the recovery of post-infarction patients.

DEVELOPMENT OF ATHEROSCLEROSIS

The Process

Autopsy examination of the coronary arteries of soldiers (whose average age was 22 years) killed in the Korean and Vietnamese conflicts showed evidence of significant atherosclerotic coronary artery disease (60% and 45% respectively). In the case of the Vietnam data, approximately 5% of those studied had at least one of the three major coronary arteries almost completely occluded or all three vessels involved to a significant degree. These data clearly demonstrate that atherosclerosis is not just a disease of the aged but is manifest early in life.

One of the major efforts in the United States to trace the development of atherosclerosis was begun in 1947 under the direction of the International Atherosclerosis Project. Researchers in this project collected approximately 30,000 aortas and coronary arteries from around the world and made cross-sectional analyses of subjects from birth to age 70. From the data, the pathologic process of atherosclerosis was established as follows [27]:

1. Below age 10:   Fatty streaks first appear in the aorta as the result of *lipid* deposition in the arterial intima (lining). This is considered benign, since it appears to occur in populations of children all around the world, regardless of diet, exercise level, or genetic background.

2. Age 10 to 20:   Fatty deposits begin to appear with increasing frequency in the coronary arteries themselves. This occurs particularly in Western populations.

3. Age 20 to 40:   The lipid materials continue to build up in the arterial wall until age 35 or 40, when they begin to change into **fibrous plaque** and become covered by fibrous scars. Most authorities feel that this development of fibrous plaque marks the point of no return: once plaque formation occurs, the process appears to be irreversible. The process can be somewhat arrested, but the scars will not disappear, as do the fatty streaks.

4. Age 40 and beyond: Finally, the areas of fibrous plaque develop into more complicated lesions involving further lipid deposition, thrombus formation, and eventual death of the tissue beyond the clot.

During the last 30 years, both epidemiological and experimental findings have made it increasingly clear that any one of a number of factors, possibly acting alone or in combination with other factors, can initiate the atherosclerotic process. The pieces of the puzzle are finally coming together. For example, improved understanding of the underlying mechanisms of lesion formation now enables scientists to link together the "lipid infiltration hypothesis" and the "endothelial injury–platelet aggregation hypothesis" [26]. More recently (1970s), the development of the "monoclonal cell proliferation theory" has further enhanced our understanding of the progressive pathologic process of atherosclerosis and has added a new dimension for exploration [3].

Multiple Risk Factor Theory

The most widely accepted theory concerning the development of atherosclerosis is the Multiple Risk Factor Theory. Epidemiologic research points towards a "multifactorial cause," involving certain factors or combinations of factors, as being responsible for increasing one's risk of the disease developing [25]. Some of the factors are statistically more strongly associated with the premature development of atherosclerosis and are identified as *primary risk factors;* others, less strongly associated, are considered as *secondary risk factors.* The following are considered *primary risk factors:*

1. Hypertension (high blood pressure)
2. Hyperlipidemia (abnormally high levels of serum triglyceride and/or serum cholesterol in circulating blood)
3. Cigarette smoking (See Figure 2-3.)

Following closely behind and not necessarily listed in order of importance are these *secondary risk factors:*

4. Obesity

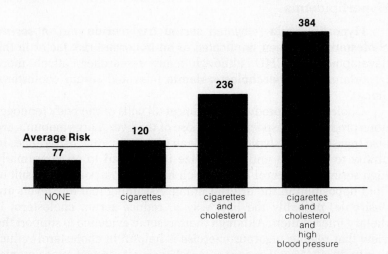

Figure 2-3. The danger of heart attack increases with the number of risk factors present. For purposes of illustration, the chart uses an abnormal blood pressure level of 180 systolic and a cholesterol level of 310 in a 45-year-old man. (Data from the Framingham, Mass., Heart Study. ©American Heart Association. Reprinted with permission.)

5. Sedentary living habits
6. Psychological or emotional stress
7. *Glucose* intolerance (diabetes mellitus)
8. Positive family history of heart disease
9. Sex (male)
10. Age

Hypertension

Hypertension (high blood pressure), salt intake, and obesity are all interrelated [7]. Except in extreme cases, blood pressure can be reduced by the control of salt intake, diet, weight, and exercise. In extreme cases, drug therapy become necessary and is effective. It is alarming that medical researchers are seeing higher blood pressures in American children today than ih the past. Although it is well known that blood pressure tends to increase with age, there is no reason to accept values higher than those listed:

Less than 5 years:	120/80
Five to 10 years:	135/85
Adolescent:	140/85
Adult:	145/90

Hyperlipidemia

Hyperlipidemia (elevated **serum triglyceride** and/or **serum cholesterol**) has been implicated as an important risk factor in the development of CHD, although many researchers attach more importance to **hypercholesterolemia** (elevated serum cholesterol alone).

Cholesterol is produced by almost all cells of the body (endogenous production), especially by those of the liver. Large amounts are also ingested in the typical American diet. Individual differences in ability to transport and metabolize it may lead to an abnormally high serum cholesterol level, which has been purported to result in lipid deposition in the arterial lining. Assuming that low levels are desirable, probably the best way to reduce serum cholesterol is dietary intervention. Although there is some evidence to support the view that regular vigorous exercise is helpful in cholesterol reduction [9, 10, 13, 20, 22], recent research, using improved experimental design, suggests that exercise effectively reduces only the triglyceride component of blood lipids [16]. It is possible that there is a cholesterol lowering effect specific to some individuals only. However, for the present and until research clearly defines the role of cholesterol in the development of CHD, it seems prudent to maintain levels below 165 and 200 milligrams of cholesterol per 100 milliliters of blood in children and adults, respectively. Cholesterol intake should not be restricted in children during their first year or so as it is important in the development of some of the components of the nervous system.

It now appears that the manner in which cholesterol travels in the bloodstream might be more important than its serum level. The major blood lipids, including cholesterol and triglyceride, are insoluble in plasma and must combine with plasma proteins to achieve solubility (hence the name *lipoproteins*). The four major lipoprotein classes are chylomicrons, very low-density lipoproteins (VLDL), **low-density lipoproteins (LDL)**, and **high-density lipoproteins (HDL)**.

Chylomicrons are composed primarily of triglyceride. They originate in the intestine from dietary fat and are metabolized rapidly in the bloodstream. VLDL is the main carrier of triglyceride and is produced primarily in the liver and small intestine. It is degraded in the blood fairly rapidly and eventually becomes LDL. LDL consists of about 60% to 75% cholesterol and is the major carrier of cholesterol to the cells.

Both the liver and the small intestine are involved in the production of HDL. When secreted directly from these organs, HDL is an immature sort of empty biconcave sac. During its maturation, it becomes spherical as its central portion fills with cholesterol. HDL is thought to assist in cholesterol removal from the tissue with the help of an enzyme called LCAT [12, 19].

Another theory considers the possibility that HDL might also inhibit the deposition of LDL in arterial cells by interfering with the cholesterol binding sites. Further investigation will be necessary to define accurately the exact biochemical mechanism responsible for the apparent cholesterol scavenging activity of HDL. Although present evidence suggests the occurrence of a "reverse cholesterol transport," and although epidemiologic studies suggest that high levels of HDL protect against CV disease, the anti-atherogenic effect of the HDL mechanism has not been clearly established [18].

After the adolescent years HDL levels fall from about 55 to about 45 milligrams per 100 milliliters of blood and remain there until beyond age 50. From epidemiologic evidence, it appears that HDL levels of approximately 55% or higher are necessary to prevent premature CHD.

Triglyceride is not ingested directly, as is cholesterol, but is synthesized within the body during carbohydrate and fat metabolism. Although dietary intervention quite effectively keeps the triglyceride level below the 150 milligrams per 100 milliliters of blood recommended by the National Institutes of Health, regular vigorous physical activity has been proven an equally effective method of triglyceride control in some people [16].

Cigarette Smoking

Cigarette smoking is one of the most physiologically damaging human habits, for it plays a significant role in the long-term development of many degenerative disorders. Smoking only one pack per day is sufficient to increase the risk of myocardial infarction three times over that of a nonsmoker. Smoking has also been shown to decrease levels of serum HDL [6]. It is regrettable to view the waste caused by so insignificant and useless an act as cigarette smoking.

Secondary Risk Factors

Of the secondary risk factors, all except sex, age and positive family history of CHD can be eliminated completely, reduced significantly, or controlled adequately.

Monoclonal Cell Proliferation Theory

Since the early 1970s, a growing body of information has become available that suggests that atherosclerosis might originate from a single mutated cell in the inner layer of an artery wall. This hypothesis, the monoclonal cell proliferation theory, comes largely from the work of Dr. Earl Benditt of the University of Washington Medical School. Dr. Benditt and co-workers [3], using an electron microscope, have been able to observe the development of an atherosclerotic lesion. They have described its stages as follows:

1. Initially, for unknown reasons, a mutation occurs in a smooth muscle cell of an artery wall (media layer), and the cell divides.
2. The daughter cell migrates into the innermost layer (the intima). This layer is normally populated by only a few cells.
3. For unknown reasons, the daughter cell proliferates and produces a mass of cells, causing a thickening of the intima and eventually resulting in a lumpy plaque.
4. Finally, there is the complication stage, in which a tendency of the cells to degenerate is seen and the lesions composed of more degenerating cells ulcerate.

It is interesting to note that electron microscopy does not support the cholesterol insudation theory (lipid infiltration hypothesis), because very little lipid is seen in the early stages of an atherosclerotic lesion [3]. The cholesterol that is eventually found in the debris can be traced to one of two sources.

1. Cholesterol can be produced endogenously by the proliferating cells.
2. Cholesterol precipitation from the serum is thought to occur because of an electrical attraction of the cholesterol molecule to ions within the lesion, independent of the level of serum cholesterol [21].

It should be pointed out that this does not necessarily preclude cholesterol from being an important factor in the development of atherosclerosis. For example, it is known that cholesterol epoxide is capable of producing connective-tissue tumors in rats and mice [3]. This mutagenic agent is also found in people with high serum cholesterol. Therefore, it is possible that cholesterol has been correctly identified as a villian but for the wrong reasons.

Whatever its explanatory merits, the monoclonal cell proliferation theory provides a new framework in which questions regarding the causes of the mutation of the original cell can be pursued.

OTHER HEART DISORDERS

Although the heart disorders that will be described are no less important than those previously mentioned, they occur less frequently and with the exception of rheumatic heart disease, are not preventable.

Congenital Defects

Congenital defects are abnormalities that are present at birth as a result of some genetic disturbance or prenatal developmental accident. Examples are atrial and ventricular septal defects produced by the failure of the heart to make postnatal adaptive changes from fetal circulation to normal circulation, coarctation of the aorta (an obstructive abnormality), and circulatory shunt disorders relating to the failure of certain fetal vessels to close at birth. Although exercise per se cannot remove these defects, psychological outlook and physiologic condition can be improved in those for whom exercise is not contraindicated. Patients with these defects must be handled individually with regard to the level of exercise that can be tolerated.

Valvular Lesions

Abnormalities of the heart valves can (1) occur congenitally, (2) result from some infectious disease, or (3) develop over the years as a result of wear and tear and mineral deposition in the valve leaflets. Some are pathologically significant and others are not. The problems associated with these types of disorders are usually twofold. First, if a valve fails to close properly, there is a backward flow **(retrograde murmur)** of blood into the chamber from which it came. This produces a volume overload and means that the affected chamber has to compensate to keep up. The defective valve is said to be *incompetent.* Second, in obstructive valvular disease, the improper formation or operation of a valve often obstructs flow through the orifice—a problem known as **stenosis.** In this case, emptying pressures higher than normal must be generated within the chamber. The usual result is pathologic enlargement (disproportionate change in the length-width ratio of myocardial cells) of that chamber (hypertrophy). It is not uncommon for a valve to become both incompetent and stenotic.

Initially, these disorders are clinically detected as abnormal heart sounds *(murmurs)* when a physician listens to the heart (auscultation). Since the 1950s, the more serious valvular lesions have been investigated by invasive techniques such as cardiac catheterization. In this procedure, tiny tubes (catheters) are threaded through vessels in the arms or legs and inserted into the chambers of the heart. Pressures in the various heart chambers can then be measured during the different phases of the cardiac cycle, and the degree of valvular incompetence can be evaluated. Use of dyes and X-ray movie photography enables physicians to assess the seriousness of a valvular lesion by observation of a diseased valve and the related blood flow patterns through the heart. Fortunately, many of the more serious problems can be corrected surgically, with the patient returning to an almost normal life-style after a short convalescent period.

In the past, physicians tended to discourage physical activity for people with heart murmurs. Unfortunately, this advice produced an unnecessarily large number of "cardiac cripples." Except in cases of relatively severe mitral or aortic stenosis, in which the risk of sudden death from exercise is high, more enlightened physicians no longer restrict activity levels because of heart murmurs. Instead, they usually encourage each individual to engage in almost any activity and allow the condition to become self-limiting. In other words, when the circulatory demands of an activity become so severe that the heart cannot pump an adequate amount of blood, fatigue ensues and the individual slows the pace or stops to rest of his or her own accord.

There is no good evidence that exercise can improve the functional ability of an incompetent or stenotic valve. However, exercise-induced bradycardia (decreased heart rate), compensation of the myocardium, and peripheral muscular adaptation are known to reduce cardiac work for a given level of activity. Any adaptation that can decrease cardiac work must be viewed as a beneficial response.

Disorders of Rhythm

Rhythmic disturbances, many of which are relatively harmless, frequently occur in apparently healthy individuals. They are manifest in the form of an unexplained excessively rapid heart rate (tachycardia), extra (ectopic) beats, or skipped beats. Clinical diagnosis can explain some of the abnormalities, but many are transient, occurring in the absence of any pathologic condition, and are therefore inexplicable. Excessive fatigue, chronic stress, overuse of caffeine and nicotine, and too little exercise have been implicated, however.

Mild cases of rhythmic dysfunction can be controlled by drug therapy using quinidine, propanolol, or similar medication. More severe disorders require surgical implantation of artificial pacemaker devices.

Rheumatic Heart Disease

Although **rheumatic heart disease** is generally preventable, it afflicts 100,000 children and 1,750,000 adults. It is caused by rheumatic fever—usually thought of as a childhood disease because it most frequently strikes between the ages of 5 and 15. This disease is always preceded by a streptococcal infection, usually a sore throat. If it is allowed to go untreated, permanent damage to the heart valves is likely to occur.

Rheumatic heart disease not only can shorten life, it can seriously reduce the quality of life. Although mortality from this disease has declined sharply since 1940, the incidence rates remain too high for a preventable disease. The first step toward prevention is identification of the streptococcal infection followed by effective treatment using penicillin or its substitutes for penicillin sensitive patients.

PREVENTIVE MEASURES IN CHD

There is general agreement among the medical community that the premature development of CHD can, to a large degree, be prevented in many people. Once it has progressed to the stage of fibrous plaque formation, the prospects for reversal are gloomy. Not to destroy all hope, however, there are a few reports of success in reversing the process using exercise, diet, and sometimes drug therapy [17, 23, 24]. If further research supports these claims, the current position on irreversibility of the process will have to be altered.

At the present time prevention of premature CHD appears to rest with the early identification of the coronary-prone individual and subsequent control of the risk factors already described in this chapter. After reviewing several risk factor modification programs, Stamler reports that real progress is being made in modifying risk factors [25].

Even so, it should be pointed out that it is not presently known whether the reduction of risk factors in persons without overt CHD will prevent its early development. Furthermore, there is no convincing evidence that changing the coronary risk profile in those individuals identified as high risk or those diagnosed as having CHD will prevent the development or alter the course of the disease.

Experimental research is underway to help answer questions like these. One example is the Multiple Risk Factor Intervention Trial (MRFIT). This study is designed to determine if a 6-year program for decreasing three major coronary risk factors will decrease the mortality from CHD among men of above average risks. Data collection on 12,886 men began in 1976 and is due to be completed in 1982. Until such time as a definitive body of evidence exists, risk factors that can be controlled, such as high blood pressure, obesity, hyperlipidemia, high anxiety levels, and excessive sodium intake, should be kept within acceptable limits.

The Role of Diet

If one accepts the hypothesis that hyperlipidemia is a major risk factor and that reduction of the level or number of risk factors will reduce the occurrence of CHD, then examination of the methods by which blood lipids may be normalized becomes important. Investigators have reported that several dietary components including total energy intake (calories), alcohol, carbohydrate, dietary cholesterol, and fat affect HDL levels. However, results from different studies have been inconsistent, mainly because of the many variables that cannot be controlled and that may confound the associations between diet and changes in HDL level [2].

Several studies have shown that when a high percentage of the diet is supplied by carbohydrate, a modest decrease in HDL results. The effects of dietary fat on HDL level are less consistent. In studies of dietary influence on HDL, the most consistent and strongest association has been between alcohol intake and HDL. These studies have repeatedly demonstrated that moderate use of alcohol increases HDL levels. Whether or not this statistically significant increase [8] represents a biologically significant elevation is yet to be determined.

In view of these findings relative to diet and alcohol, it would appear that eating a normal balanced diet in the proportions recommended by the Senate Select Committee on Nutrition and Human Needs remains sound advice for the prevention of premature CHD. (See Chapter 6, p. 117.) One should, however, be cautious about using alcohol to elevate HDL. At this time it is not recommended that nondrinkers begin using alcohol to raise HDL levels. No experimental studies establishing the biological benefits of such a procedure have been reported, and the potential for socioeconomic trauma that is associated with alcohol abuse cannot be ignored. On the other hand, those who use alcohol moderately probably should not be advised to discontinue, at least not for medical reasons. These people should be aware, however, that heavy usage unquestionably enhances the development of several severe cardiovascular problems and other health hazards [14, 15].

The Role of Exercise

For years many have claimed that vigorous exercise throughout life is a major deterrent to the development of CHD. A former president of the American Medical Joggers Association even went so far as to claim that people who train for and complete marathons do not develop CHD. He was challenged by colleagues from around the world, and evidence from autopsy findings has been presented which has dispelled the myth that marathon running provides immunity to CHD. Although the incidence is lower in people who adopt the life-style of the marathon runner, whether it is accurate to infer that running (exercise) is responsible for this phenomenon or whether these individuals select this most strenuous type of exercise because of some genetic predisposition remains highly controversial.

Moderate exercise does appear to exert a positive influence on several risk factors. Evidence is now convincing that exercise increases the level of HDL cholesterol, which is interpreted as a protective mechanism against lipid deposition in blood vessel walls [11, 29, 30]. Regular exercise is also one of the best methods for decreasing the level of blood triglyceride. It has also been proven useful in reducing blood pressure in some individuals, and its value in weight management is well documented. Furthermore, regular exercise is effective in reducing emotional stress and the amount of insulin required by diabetics. Undoubtedly exercise is valuable therapy for reducing risk factors.

Finally, the questions of how much one should exercise to reduce the risk of CHD and whether risk factor reduction does, in fact, reduce risk of premature CHD are as yet unanswered. Present opinions range from as little as 15 minutes triweekly to as much as 6 miles or 1 hour of daily continuous running at a good pace if significant protection against CHD is to occur. Until well-controlled scientific research provides an answer, it should be assumed that the benefit derived is generally proportional to the exercise input. This concept is discussed more fully in Chapters 3 and 4.

CARDIAC REHABILITATION

If preventive measures have been begun too late and a cardiac incident occurs, one finds a certain comfort in the knowledge that modern medical technology can, in many cases, enable a patient to be rehabilitated. Coronary bypass surgery for reconstructing occluded arteries, valve replacement by open-heart surgery, and pacemaker implants are important achievements that have become fairly common during the past decade.

The medical literature is saturated with reports of the therapeutic value of exercise as one mode of rehabilitating patients predisposed to CHD. With few exceptions, cardiac patients respond to physical training in much the same manner as do athletes. In addition to reconditioning the heart, exercise reconditions the skeletal muscles, which some consider to be of equal benefit. Since post-training heart rate and blood pressure are both lower at comparable work levels, cardiac work is reduced and functional cardiac reserve power is thereby increased [4, 28].

Although many heart attack victims have made remarkable recoveries through rehabilitative efforts involving changes in lifestyle, the reader should be aware that not all individuals respond well to physical training. Dr. John Cantwell, co-director of Cardiac Rehabilitation of Georgia Baptist Hospital, has outlined characteristics of a highly trainable postinfarction patient as follows [5]:

1. Less than 55 years old
2. Uncomplicated inferior myocardial infarction
3. Able to achieve greater than 85% of age-predicted maximum heart rate during an exercise test
4. Less than 20% body fat
5. Nonsmoker or ex-smoker
6. Former athlete (physically well-trained individual)

It is interesting to note that half of the items listed are somewhat controllable, and that one (number 6) suggests the value of a physically active adolescence and young adulthood.

REFERENCES

1. American Heart Association. *Heart facts 1980.* Dallas: American Heart Association, 1980.
2. American Society for Clinical Nutrition. Symposium: Report on the task force on the evidence relating six dietary factors to the nation's health. *The American Journal of Clinical Nutrition* 32 (12):2621-2748, 1979 (suppl.).
3. Benditt, E. The origin of atherosclerosis. *Scientific American* 236 (2):74-85, 1977.
4. Bruce, R. A. Principles of exercise testing. In *Exercise testing and exercise training in coronary heart disease,* edited by J. P. Naughton and H. K. Hellerstein. New York: Academic Press, 1973.
5. Cantwell, J. D. Presentation, Quinton Exercise Stress Testing Seminar, Atlanta, Georgia, January 1978.
6. Criqui, M. H.; Wallace, R. B.; Heiss, G.; Mishkel, M.; Schonfeld, G.; and Jones, G. T. L. Cigarette smoking and plasma high density lipoprotein cholesterol. *Circulation* 62 (suppl. IV):70-76, 1980.
7. Dustan, H. P. Research contributions toward prevention of cardiovascular disease: Research related to the underlying mechanisms in hypertension. *Circulation* 60 (7):1566-1568, 1979.
8. Ernst, N.; Fisher, M.; Smith, W.; Gordon, T.; Rifkind, B. M.; Little, J. A.; Mishkel, M. A.; and Williams, O. D. The association of plasma high density lipoprotein cholesterol with dietary intake and alcohol consumption. *Circulation* 62 (suppl. IV):41-52, 1980.
9. Fox, S. M., and Haskell, W. L. Physical activity and the prevention of heart disease. *Bulletin of the New York Academy of Medicine,* 2d series 44:950, August 1968.
10. Gustafson, A. Effect of training on blood lipids. In *Coronary heart disease and physical fitness,* edited by O. A. Larsen and R. O. Malmborg. Baltimore: University Park Press, 1971.
11. Hartung, G. H.; Foreyt, J. P.; Mitchell, R. E.; Vlasek, I.; and Gotto, A. M. Relation of diet to high-density-lipoprotein cholesterol in middle-age

marathon runners, joggers, and inactive men. *The New England Journal of Medicine* 302 (7):357–361, 1980.

12. Havel, R. J. High-density lipoproteins, cholesterol transport, and coronary heart disease. *Circulation* 60 (1):1–3, 1979.

13. Joseph, J. J., and Bena, L. L. Cholesterol reduction—a long term intense exercise program. *Journal of Sports Medicine and Physical Fitness* 17 (2):163–168, 1977.

14. Klatsky, A. L. Alcohol and cardiovascular disorders. *Primary Cardiology* 5 (9):86–95, 1979.

15. Klatsky, A. L. Alcohol and cardiovascular disorders. *Primary Cardiology* 5(10):76–83, 1979.

16. Lampman, R. M.; Santinga, J. T.; Bassett, D. R.; Mercer, N.; Block, W. D.; Flora, J. D.; Foss, M. D.; and Thorland, W. G. Effectiveness of unsupervised and supervised high intensity physical training in normalizing serum lipids in men with type IV hyperlipoproteinemia. *Circulation* 57 (1):172–180, 1978.

17. Leonard, J. N.; Hofer, J. L.; and Pritikin, N. *Live longer now.* New York: Grosset and Dunlap, 1974.

18. Levy, R. I., and Rifkind, B. M. The structure, function and metabolism of high-density lipoproteins: A status report. *Circulation* 62 (suppl. IV):4–8, 1980.

19. Lindgren, F. T., ed. *Symposium: High density lipoproteins (HDL).* Champaign, Illinois: American Oil Chemists' Society, 1979.

20. Milesis, C. A. Effects of metered physical training on serum lipids of adult men. *Journal of Sports Medicine and Physical Fitness* 14:8–13, 1974.

21. Passwater, R. *Supernutrition for healthy hearts.* New York: Dial Press, 1977.

22. Pollack, M. J.; Tiffany, J.; Gettman, L.; Janeway, R.; and Loftland, H. B. Effects of frequency of training on serum lipids, cardiovascular function and body composition. In *Exercise and fitness,* edited by D. B. Frunks. Chicago: Athletic Institute, 1969.

23. Pritikin, N., and McGrady, P. M., Jr. *The Pritikin program for diet and exercise.* New York: Bantam Books, 1980.

24. Schettler, G.; Goto, Y.; Hata, Y.; and Klose, G., eds. *Atherosclerosis IV.* New York: Springer-Verlag, 1977.

25. Stamler, J. Research related to risk factors. *Circulation* 60 (7):1575–1587, 1979.

26. Steinberg, D. Research related to underlying mechanisms in atherosclerosis. *Circulation* 60 (7):1559–1565, 1979.

27. Strong, W. B. The natural history and pathogenesis of atherosclerosis: Pediatric aspects. Presented at the Southeast Regional Meeting of the American College of Sports Medicine, Columbia, South Carolina, November 1975.

28. Wenger, N. K. Research related to rehabilitation. *Circulation* 60 (7):1636–1639, 1979.

29. Wood, P. D., and Haskell, W. L. The effect of exercise on plasma high density lipoproteins. *Lipids* 14 (4):417–427, 1979.

30. Wood, P. D.; Haskell, W. L.; Stern, M. P.; Lewis, S.; and Perry, C. Plasma lipoprotein distribution in male and female runners. *Annals of the New York Academy of Sciences* 301:748–763, 1977.

KEY TERMS
Asymptomatic (p. 28)
Maximum heart rate range (p. 33)
MET (p. 35)
Stress test (p. 26)
Symptomatic (p. 28)

BEHAVIORAL OBJECTIVES
Upon completion of this chapter, the student should be able to:
1. Define the key terms listed above.
2. Outline the eight steps to be taken in formulating an exercise prescription.
3. Select and self-administer a suitable test for classification of the functional capacity of the circulorespiratory (CR) system.
4. Describe the precautions that should be followed with respect to engaging in an exercise program.
5. Determine his or her target heart rate for training.
6. Determine the energy cost in Calories and in METS of an activity when the intensity, duration, and body weight of the participant are provided.

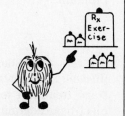

Although strenuous physical activity is not a panacea for all the ills of humankind, it is widely accepted that a regular program of vigorous, rhythmic exercise enhances the quality of life by increasing the physical capability for work and play [3]. On the basis of current evidence, it is not justifiable to conclude that exercise alone is the key to the prevention of heart disease [1]. But each year the data become increasingly favorable in support of continued vigorous physical activity throughout life as a valuable adjunct to the elimination of certain risk factors, such as cigarette smoking, high blood pressure, and high blood lipids, in reducing the probability that coronary heart disease will develop.

While it has been established that exercise is valuable in the rehabilitation of individuals who have certain types of cardiovascular disease [5], and even though the literature supports exercise as a strong contributor to the prevention of atherosclerotic coronary artery disease, one should be cautious of engaging in an unsupervised vigorous program of physical training. Does this mean that exercise is dangerous? Not necessarily. For persons under age 35 who are subject to none of the primary risk factors, the probability of bodily damage from sensible physical exercise is so remote that it can be disregarded. However, there are individuals who could benefit greatly from certain types of exercise regimens at specified tolerance levels but for whom engagement in more strenuous activity might be extremely hazardous or even fatal. There are also a few for whom almost any level of exercise is so dangerous that the risks of mortality far outweigh any small benefits to be gained. These people should not exercise.

The problem, then, is to determine for each individual the amount of risk that is involved, the kind of program that is in order, and the level of exercise that can safely be tolerated. The solution to the problem lies in the analysis of data collected during a procedure designed to evaluate the functional capacity of an individual. This procedure, commonly called a **stress test** or a *graded exercise test,* should be performed prior to participation in any strenuous exercise program.

THE STRESS TEST

A stress test usually consists either of riding a stationary bicycle (bicycle ergometer) or of walking and/or running during a multistage treadmill test (see Figure 3-1) while one's blood pressure, electrocardiogram (ECG), and general response to exercise are

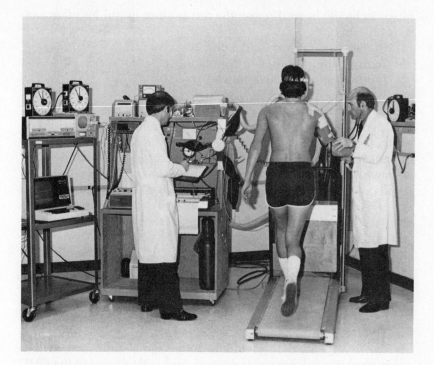

Figure 3-1. Treadmill stress test.

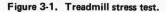

monitored by a physician. In either case, the work load is gradually increased in a stepwise fashion until (1) a predetermined target heart rate is attained; (2) the person can no longer continue; or (3) symptoms of cardiovascular disease are observed, which dictate that the test be terminated. The primary purpose of the test, when directed by a physician, is to identify the presence of silent ischemic heart disease by means of the ECG in the absence of clinical symptoms. Although the testing of persons under age 35 without significant risk factors is not likely to identify more than one case in a hundred, ischemic responses can be expected with greater frequency as age increases. In addition to revealing the presence of

latent ischemic heart disease, the test is often useful for other reasons [3]:
1. To evaluate cardiovascular functional capacity
2. To evaluate responses to conditioning
3. To increase individual motivation

Who Should Have a Stress Test?

Ideally, all who plan to engage in strenuous exercise would be well advised to take a physician-administered stress test first. Even in apparently healthy, **asymptomatic,** young adults, it can be valuable to establish an ECG base line, which can be compared with the results of some future test if the question of abnormality should arise. Realistically, however, graded exercise tests are quite expensive, and testing sites are often not conveniently located for those who might desire to be tested. Fortunately, people who are able to exercise safely can usually be identified with proper screening during a routine medical examination, including a review of family history of heart disease and a resting ECG. On the basis of the findings of such examinations, the American College of Sports Medicine Committee on Exercise and Stress Testing recommends that candidates for exercise be classified and advised as follows [1]:
1. For asymptomatic individuals under age 35 with no previous history of cardiovascular disease, and without any of the CHD primary risk factors, the risk involved in the increase of habitual physical activity is low enough that special medical clearance is not required. If questionable symptoms develop or if this individual has not had a medical examination during the previous two years, consultation with a physician seems to be the wise and prudent course before proceeding with an exercise program.
2. For those 35 years of age or younger who have had or who show evidence of cardiovascular disease or who have significant combinations of positive family history of cardiovascular disease, elevated blood pressure (hypertension), hyperlipidemia, diabetes mellitus, cigarette smoking, or obesity, medical clearance is highly recommended prior to any significant increase in physical activity level.
3. Regardless of health status, all persons above age 35 are advised to receive medical clearance before they increase activity levels. Furthermore, it is advised that all persons over age 35 and all those under age 35 who are either high risk or **symptomatic** take an ECG-monitored graded exercise test conducted

under the supervision of a qualified physician prior to any major increases in exercise.

GUIDELINES FOR THE EXERCISE PRESCRIPTION

Best results from any training program are assured when the exercise regimen is prepared on scientifically sound principles and is based on the results of a preliminary evaluation of the subject's circulorespiratory (CR) function, health, interests, motor proficiency, and available facilities [2]. Eight steps are easily identifiable in the development of an individualized exercise prescription (EP). They are (1) medical clearance, (2) identification of a personal fitness goal, (3) some form of CR fitness evaluation (e.g., Cooper's Twelve-Minute Run, Harvard Step Test), (4) selection of a training style or styles, (5) establishment of exercise frequency, (6) establishment of exercise intensity, (7) determination of the duration of each exercise session, and (8) periodic reevaluation of CR fitness and program adjustment if necessary.

Medical Clearance

If the presence of CHD risk factors, overt symptoms of cardiac impairment, or age suggests that exercise might not be well tolerated, medical clearance should be sought before an individual engages in any significant increase in physical activity. If, however, there are no contraindications to physical activity, it is not hazardous for most people to develop and engage in their own individualized exercise program.

Goal Identification

Because exercise benefits are closely related to the type of training one employs, it is imperative that the desired level of fitness be identified. Equally important is the definition of the desired type of fitness (e.g., strength, CR endurance, speed). Obviously, those who want to run marathons require different styles and levels of training from those who prefer to participate in recreational sports activities that utilize different muscle groups and demand lower levels of CR endurance.

Circulorespiratory Fitness Evaluation

Unless one falls into a category that requires a physician-administered stress test, less sophisticated, self-administered tests are very helpful in estimating CR fitness levels. Two such tests are

Cooper's Twelve-Minute Run and the Harvard Step Test. These tests are described in Laboratory Sessions 5 and 6 and can be used to determine the appropriate initial training stimulus.

Selection of a Training Style and Exercise Type

Selection of the type of exercise and the training style is critical to the success of an exercise program for at least two reasons. First, the appropriateness of these two factors determines whether or not the training results will be consistent with the goals that have been identified. Second, the style must provide a pleasant training experience or the long-term commitment to exercise is not likely to persist. It is wise to vary both training style and surroundings to relieve the boredom that so often sets in when the same routine is followed over an extended period.

The most basic principle behind any type of training is that it should overload the body beyond normal daily demands. Second, training has a specificity effect: only the body part that is overloaded improves, and the improvement is specific to the type of exercise used. Because of this, several types of exercise are available. It is important to know the training effect expected from each type. To become physically fit, one needs to devise a program that stresses work in circulorespiratory endurance, muscular endurance, strength, and flexibility. Chapter 4 provides more detailed information about training styles and their effects.

CIRCULORESPIRATORY ENDURANCE

If a training regimen were to contain only one type of exercise, then one that develops circulorespiratory endurance would be preferable. Running, swimming, and cycling are three commonly chosen activities used to develop *aerobic power.* These types of movements, when vigorously engaged in, overload the oxygen-transport system and result in an increase in circulorespiratory endurance. Any activity that involves the large-muscle groups of the body in continuous, rhythmic, *dynamic contraction* is satisfactory.

MUSCULAR STRENGTH AND ENDURANCE

It is generally accepted that methods of developing strength and methods of developing endurance lie at opposite ends of a continuum. Strength is best developed by high-resistance, low-repetition exercises, which are dynamic. On the other hand, to improve endurance, either circulorespiratory or muscular, one must alter the traditional strength-training procedure by adding further repetitions.

If one wants to develop both strength and muscular endurance, strength is usually the initial concern until the desired level is achieved. Then the regimen is altered to provide increased endurance. (See Chapter 4.)

Isometric exercise has been proved effective in increasing strength; however, the authors have two serious reservations about recommending it. First, research indicates that *isometric contraction* appears to enhance strength most at the angle at which contraction is performed. Second, static strains are potentially dangerous to poorly conditioned individuals and persons with compromised cardiovascular function. At any rate, neither isometric nor dynamic exercise is effective in the improvement of circulorespiratory endurance.

FLEXIBILITY AND RELAXATION ACTIVITIES

As a result of inactivity or aging, the range of motion in joints progressively decreases. Maintaining flexibility is highly desirable and can be achieved by means of slow stretching movements. A posture at the limit of one's range of motion should be held momentarily, then followed by a further effort to stretch the joint and the corresponding muscle groups. Rapid, forced, ballistic bouncing is not recommended because tissue damage might occur. It has been suggested that this type of bouncing might even be detrimental to flexibility, owing to muscular response to the *stretch reflex*. Additional information on flexibility can be found in Chapter 5.

In recent years, more emphasis has been placed on relaxation activities. (See Chapter 7.) The key lies in identifying the source of muscular tension. Relaxation is then achieved by vigorous contraction of that particular muscle group while breathing freely, after which a conscious attempt at complete muscular relaxation is made. These exercises are most effectively used during the warm-up and cool-down periods of an exercise session [1].

Training Frequency, Intensity, and Duration

It is important to understand that training frequency, intensity, and duration are interrelated in the exercise prescription. Even if one variable is altered, a concomitant adjustment in one or both of the remaining variables can be made to produce the same result. Thus, these variables can be manipulated to prevent injury in the initial stage of a regimen and to ward off boredom or to increase the training stimulus during some later stage.

When planning an exercise program, one does well to remember that the initial improvement in sedentary individuals generally occurs in proportion to the amount of work accomplished. Later, as the physical condition improves, further increases in the work load elicit diminished gains in relation to work input. This necessitates periodic revisions of the exercise prescription if continued improvement is desired. At some point, however, when improvement is no longer the goal, the program changes to one of maintenance. Thus, when one is faced with decisions about how often (frequency), how long (duration), and how hard (intensity) the exercise program should be, two major criteria should be kept in mind: first, the entry level of the participant, and second, the goals and how soon they must be achieved.

It appears that, except for very deconditioned people, fewer than three workouts per week is not sufficient to produce measurable training benefits. Three workouts per week has been demonstrated to be beneficial for most sedentary persons. After a moderate level of training has been attained, however, the frequency usually must be increased if continued improvement is to be observed. Therefore, after the initial triweekly period, and except in the case of those who are preparing for world class competition, training frequency should be increased to four or five weekly sessions interspaced by occasional rest days. The rest days allow the body to rebuild tissues that inevitably become worn and injured, and they offer psychological relief to those who become bored with the regularity of the regimen.

The question often arises as to how the work sessions should be spaced when there are fewer than five per week. Participants have traditionally been advised to space training sessions symmetrically on alternate days throughout the week, although conclusive scientific data are not presently available. In a study involving the placement of triweekly training sessions, no difference in improvements was found between persons who symmetrically spaced training and rest days and persons who worked for three consecutive days and rested for four [4]. Despite this evidence of improved aerobic power with nonsymmetrical spacing of training sessions, the effectiveness of exercise in the reduction of serum triglyceride levels for 24 to 36 hours after a vigorous workout appears to make symmetrical spacing more advisable.

Intensity and duration are inversely related. For the development of circulorespiratory endurance, it seems more desirable to increase the duration (within reasonable limits) at the expense of intensity, rather than vice versa, particularly in symptomatic individuals over 35 years old. The total exercise period for normal participants should be at least 20 to 30 minutes. It should include an initial 5- to 10-minute warm-up period (longer for the older and the less well conditioned) and should end with approximately 10 minutes of cool-down and relaxation activities. A minimum of 15 minutes of aerobic exercise, exclusive of warm-up and cool-down, is recommended. Twenty to 30 minutes of aerobic exercise is more desirable.

Determining the intensity of exercise is probably the most important part of an exercise prescription. Several guidelines are helpful. It must always be remembered that training effects ensue *only* if the amount of the overload (training stimulus) is greater than some minimal amount of work necessary to maintain normal physiologic function and that the level of this stimulus varies among individuals.

One of the most frequent mistakes made by those who are beginning exercise regimens is to work too hard too soon. The resultant general malaise and localized muscular soreness experienced by formerly sedentary people is often a turning off rather than a turning on to exercise. In addition, failure to allow adequate time for the musculoskeletal system to adapt to this new form of stress too often results in painful "overuse" injury that could be avoided by slowly and progressively increasing the amount of exercise as tolerance improves. There is no hurry, no deadline to meet, because we are talking about a lifetime commitment—not a crash program to develop fitness. It should also be understood that the training effect appears to be dependent, at least in part, on the total amount of work accomplished. Therefore, the initial workouts should be low intensity with musculoskeletal adaptation as the primary goal. After this initial phase, the intensity can be safely increased to 60% to 75% of the maximum heart rate range. Work at this level should produce substantial improvement within 6 to 8 months. Thereafter, the rate of improvement will likely decline. Until one becomes very well conditioned, work above this level is not well tolerated and is therefore not recommended. Translated into practical terms, one should feel fully recovered within approximately one hour after exercise. Otherwise the program is too severe [1].

Researchers have fairly well defined the threshold necessary to produce measurable gains in aerobic capacity as roughly 60% of one's **maximum heart rate range.** Just as one can train at an intensity too low to be of any benefit (i.e., below 60%), training can also be more rigorous than necessary to accomplish the desired goals. Except in the case of athletes preparing for world class competition, there is no need to train at intensities greater than 85% to 90% of one's aerobic capacity. Furthermore, too high a training level might even be hazardous to those with exercise limitations.

QUANTIFYING INTENSITY

There are several indices available to quantify the intensity of a training program. It is the wise participant who learns the technique of self-monitoring responses to the training stimulus, both during the workout as well as over the long term. Because heart rate, work load, and oxygen uptake are linearly related in the normal workout ranges, any of these is suitable for monitoring training intensity.

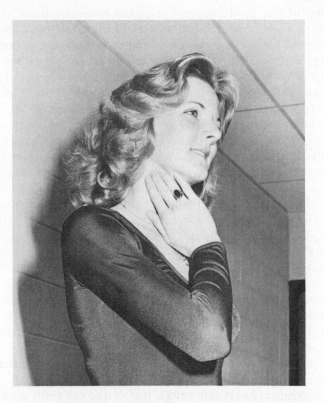

Figure 3-2. Palpation of carotid pulse.

Heart rate is the easiest to monitor and is probably used most frequently. To determine heart rate, the first and second fingers are placed lightly on the carotid artery, located in the neck (see Figure 3-2), the pulsations are counted for 10 seconds, and multiplied by 6 to find the number of beats per minute. Only one carotid should be selected for *palpation,* and the pressure should be very light to prevent stimulation of the *baroreceptors,* which reflexively reduce heart rate. In addition, if an estimate of exercise heart rate is desired, the measurement must be made during the *first 10 seconds immediately* after the cessation of the exercise.

The heart rate at which one should work can be calculated very easily (see Table 3-1) as is demonstrated in the following problem. Assume that an exercise prescription calls for work at 60% of the maximum heart rate range. Assume a maximum heart rate of 200 beats per minute (this is the predicted value for a normal 20-year-old) and a resting heart rate of 70 beats per minute. The effective or maximum heart rate range is calculated by subtracting the resting heart rate from the maximum heart rate, which gives a potential increase of 130 beats per minute. This figure is then multiplied by 0.6 (for a 60% increase), which gives 78 beats per minute and is added to the resting rate. The target heart rate for satisfying the prescribed intensity level is therefore 78 + 70 = 148 beats per minute. The resting and maximum heart rate values may change from person to person, along with the intensity; however, the procedure for calculation does not change. (See Figure 3-3.) If maximum heart rate is not known, a generally acceptable estimate can be made by subtracting one's age in years from 220.

An alternative method to the use of the heart rate as an index of circulatory stress is gaining wider acceptance among exercise physiologists and medical personnel. This method employs multiples of the resting metabolic rate (**MET**), which represent the amount of oxygen used in the performance of various activities (expressed as milliliters of oxygen consumed per kilogram of body weight per minute). One MET is approximately 3.5 ml/kg per minute. Two METs represent work requiring 7.0 ml/kg per minute, 3 METs represent 10.5 ml/kg per minute, and so on.

The maximum functional capacity of most sedentary individuals is about 8 to 10 METs, and in highly trained athletes it is about 16 to 20 METs. Accordingly, a work intensity of 4 METs represents 50% of the functional capacity of an individual whose maximum capacity is 8 METs, whereas this same load represents only 25% of the capacity of an athlete whose maximum is 16 METs. Consequently,

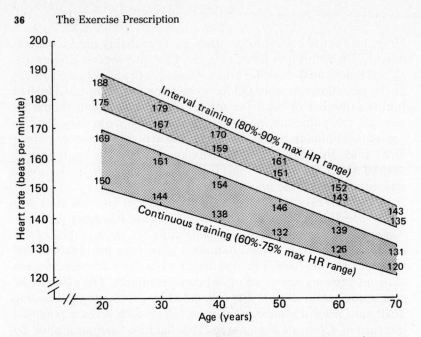

Figure 3-3. Training heart rate (HR) zones for increasing aerobic capacity. (Rates were calculated using the Karvonen formula and assuming a resting HR of 75 beats per minute and a maximum HR of 220−age.)

the intensity represented by a MET is absolute in terms of the amount of oxygen consumed but relative with respect to the functional capacity of an individual. That is to say, 8 METs might be all that one individual can tolerate, but it might tax another individual at only 50%. Some common activities along with their approximate MET values can be seen in Table 6-10.

A third method of quantifying the level of the training stimulus makes use of the number of Calories required for a particular workout. Although appropriate for any exerciser, it should be particularly attractive to those who plan to use exercise to assist in weight reduction. To use the method, one needs only to consult Table 6-10 or one similar.

Assume that the exercise prescription for a 150-pound person calls for a 200 Cal/day workout to assist in weight reduction and that the participant's exercise choice is jogging. From Table 6-10 it can be seen that jogging at 5 mph requires an energy expenditure of 0.0667 Cal/lb per minute. Multiplied by this person's body weight (150 pounds), the energy cost becomes about 10 Cal/min (0.0667 Cal/lb

TABLE 3-1
DETERMINATION OF TARGET HEART RATE FOR TRAINING

			Sample
1. Predicted maximum heart rate* (use actual rate if known)	=	(200)	200
2. Resting heart rate (end of week 1)	= −		− 70
3. Maximum heart range	=		130
4. Percentage desired for training (use 60%, 70%, 80%)	= x		x0.60
5. Multiply step 3 by step 4	=		78
6. Resting heart rate	= +		+70
7. Target heart rate for training (end of week 1)	=		148

NOTE: Periodic revision of target heart rate will become necessary as resting heart rate changes.
*If maximum heart rate is not known, a generally acceptable estimate can be made by subtracting one's age from 220. See M. Karvonen, K. Kentala, and O. Muslala, The effects of training heart rate: A longitudinal study, *Annales Medicinae Experimentalis et Biologiae Fenniae* 35:307-315, 1957.

TABLE 3-2
RECORD OF RESTING HEART RATE

	Resting Heart Rate	Target Heart Rate
End of week 1		
End of week 2		
End of week 3		
End of week 4		
End of week 8		
End of last week		

per minute × 150 lb). It follows that utilization of 200 Calories by jogging at the rate of 5 mph would require approximately 20 minutes (200 Cal ÷ 10 Cal/min).

Periodic Reevaluation

Periodic evaluation of progress is an important index to the effectiveness of the training program and to whether or not the rate of improvement is normal. Although the rate of improvement of circulorespiratory endurance is fairly predictable in normal, healthy individuals within a specific age group, it is valuable to find out if one is achieving one's goals. In addition, as fitness improves, the target heart rate for training is subject to change (i.e., a comparable stimulus is achieved at a lower training heart rate). For these reasons periodic reevaluation of circulorespiratory fitness is recommended.

DEVELOPMENT OF AN EXERCISE PRESCRIPTION

Scott and Cindy are 19-year-old college students. Their weights are only slightly above normal. They have no functional impairment, and they are not regular exercisers. Sporadic attempts at tennis, basketball, and other recreational activities leave them sore and demonstrate a decline in the physical fitness they enjoyed during their earlier years. Several of their friends are physically active and have encouraged Scott and Cindy to join them but they cannot keep up. Furthermore, they are apprehensive about their ability to recondition themselves properly. Using the steps outlined in this chapter they could proceed as follows.

Looking at the guidelines for the exercise prescription, they find themselves in a category that does not demand special medical clearance. Even so, they should use good common sense as they train and "listen to their bodies" for signals that might warrant medical advice.

Next they set their training goals. They have heard and read about the many benefits of regular exercise and they admire the self-confidence and apparent physical fitness displayed by their runner friends. Though not now possible, they would eventually like to join them in their daily 2- or 3-mile runs, which are usually covered at a pace of about 8.5 min/mile.

Having chosen this goal, they need to evaluate their present level of CR fitness so as to initiate an appropriate training stimulus. To accomplish this, Scott and Cindy self-administer the Cooper's

Twelve-Minute Run (see Laboratory Session 5) and find that they can complete only 1.3 and 1.2 miles, respectively, in the allotted time. These results indicate that their CR fitness is only fair. (See Appendix A.)

The training style most likely to help Scott and Cindy initially will be an interval approach involving brief periods of work inter-spaced with rest periods of equal length. As their exercise tolerance improves, they should work toward a continuous effort by gradually increasing the length of the work periods while decreasing the time spent resting.

Adhering to the general principle that those in average or poorer fitness categories need to train three times per week, they select Monday, Wednesday, and Friday as their training days. (Scott and Cindy might like to train 5 days per week for faster progress, but they are aware that "overuse" at any point in training, and particu-larly during the early weeks, increases the possibility for musculo-skeletal injury.) After 3 or 4 weeks they might try increasing the frequency of the workouts to 4 or 5 days per week so long as their backs, legs, ankles, and feet do not indicate ill effects.

Scott and Cindy are concerned about how intense their workout should be. Looking through an old college text, they find that they are not likely to experience any significant improvement unless they work in excess of 60% of their maximum heart rate range. Using the procedure described in Table 3-1, Scott calculates his target heart rate to be 149 beats per minute. He should not exceed 75% of his maximum heart rate range (168 beats per minute), so that the work does not become uncomfortably difficult during the relatively long periods of continuous work. Having determined this range, he should try to reach the minimum stimulus (heart rate = 149) after about 3 minutes of work. By approximately halfway through the workout he should be at 65% or 70% of his maximum heart rate range (heart rate = 155 to 162). He should approach the upper limit of the training range (heart rate = 168) by the end of the workout.

Because Cindy's resting heart rate (80 beats per minute) is higher than Scott's (70 beats per minute), her minimum target heart rate (153) will be somewhat higher, as well as her training range (153 to 171). In spite of these small differences, she must follow the same principles of training relative to target heart rate and training range that have been prescribed for Scott. This will probably mean that if Cindy and Scott wish to train together, she will have to work at a greater relative work load owing to her smaller and less efficient circulorespiratory system. That is to say, at a given running pace, a greater demand is placed on the female's CR system than on that of her male partner.

The last critical decision Scott and Cindy have to make concerns the length of each workout. Ultimately, the greater the quantity of work (to a point), the greater the benefit. However, a realistic approach must take into account their personal fitness goals as well as the time they are willing to devote to training. They must also remember that intensity, duration, and frequency are interrelated and can be manipulated in various combinations to produce the desired result. Two general principles will be helpful here: the principle of working within a training heart rate range, and the principle that about 300 Calories should be expended at the appropriate heart rate for CR benefits to accrue [2].

In the early stages (first 3 to 5 weeks) of their training regimen, they should settle for 15 to 20 minutes of triweekly walking/jogging, at least until their musculoskeletal system can endure greater stress. After they have gradually worked up to about 2 continuous miles (within the prescribed heart rate range), the speed over distance should be increased to provide the necessary overload for continuing improvement. Periodic reevaluation (every 4 to 6 months) of CR fitness is advisable to determine if the training regimen remains adequate.

Precautions

In general, apparently healthy, asymptomatic persons whose functional capacities are at least 8 METs can participate safely in an unsupervised conditioning program. For symptomatic persons, regardless of their functional capacities, or for asymptomatic persons whose functional capacities are less than 8 METs, supervised exercise programs are advised, at least until it is deemed safe for them to exercise on their own [1]. Additional precautions seem warranted as follows [3]:

1. Exercise should be avoided when it can aggravate a minor illness, injury, or infection or retard recovery from illness. Even when one simply does not feel well, exercise could be dangerous, because illness might be incipient.
2. Strenuous exercise is hazardous in unusual environmental conditions (heat and humidity), during times of emotional stress, or immediately after ingestion of a heavy meal. In these cases, the intensity must be decreased or the exercise even abandoned.
3. Cool-down periods should occur in the same environment as the exercise. In no case should one move from a cooler to a

warmer environment during a cool-down period after strenuous exercise.

4. Hot showers should be avoided during the immediate postexercise period, particularly in the over-35 age group. In rare instances, hot showers have been associated with immediate occurrence of heart attack.

Summary

In summary, the following steps appear to be reasonable when one makes a commitment to exercise throughout life:

1. Preliminary determination of individual functional capacity in relation to the degree of risk involved in exercise, with subsequent medical clearance or restriction.
2. Development of an appropriate exercise prescription, scientifically based on individual objectives, needs, functional capacity, and interests.
3. Regular, prudent participation in the prescribed regimen, with attention to safety precautions and contraindications to exercise.
4. Periodic reassessment of functional capacity in terms of adaptation to training, with subsequent adjustment of the prescription if indicated.

REFERENCES

1. American College of Sports Medicine. *Guidelines for graded-exercise testing and exercise prescription.* Philadelphia: Lea and Febiger, 1975.
2. American College of Sports Medicine. *Guidelines for graded-exercise testing and exercise prescription.* 2d ed. Philadelphia: Lea and Febiger, 1980.
3. American Heart Association. *Exercise testing and training of apparently healthy individuals: A handbook for physicians.* New York: American Heart Association, 1972.
4. Moffatt, R. J.; Stamford, B. A.; and Neill, R. D. Placement of triweekly training sessions: Importance regarding enhancement of aerobic capacity. *Research Quarterly* 48 (3):583–591, 1977.
5. Naughton, J. P., and Hellerstein, H. K., eds. *Exercise testing and exercise training in coronary heart disease.* New York: Academic Press, 1973.

CHAPTER FOUR

TRAINING PROGRAMS AND THEIR EFFECTS

KEY TERMS
Interval training (p. 46)
Jogging (p. 45)
Repetition max (RM) (p. 50)
Set (p. 50)
Specificity effect (p. 44)
Work-relief ratio (p. 46)

BEHAVIORAL OBJECTIVES
Upon completion of this chapter, the student should be able to:

1. Define the key terms listed above.
2. Differentiate between types of training programs with regard to expected benefits.
3. Develop an individualized training program for improving circulorespiratory endurance.
4. Develop an individualized training program for improving strength.
5. Describe the procedure used in circuit training.
6. List the physiological adaptations to endurance training.
7. List the physiological adaptations to strength training.
8. List six exercise-induced injuries.

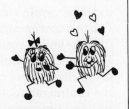

PRINCIPLES OF TRAINING

Van Huss et al. [56] list several goals that supposedly motivate people to train. Some of the more common ones are:

1. Development of physique
2. Improvement of general physical condition
3. Increase in proficiency in sports skills
4. Weight control
5. Rehabilitation from injury or disease
6. Protection from injury

The training procedures used to accomplish these ends take various forms. As was indicated in Chapter 3, one must decide what kinds of benefits are desired prior to formulation of a training program. Only after personal objectives are clearly identified can decisions regarding exercise type, frequency, and intensity be made. It is essential that individuals desiring to train understand the principal concepts basic to the development and maintenance of any training program.

First, the **specificity effect** of training, mentioned in Chapter 3, should be emphasized. This means that one benefits only in specific ways from particular kinds of training. For example, if one engages in activities that primarily involve the legs, then the arms do not benefit. Training is even more specific to limbs or muscle groups. Roberts and Alspaugh [45] clearly demonstrated this in a cycling and running experiment. Thirty-six subjects were initially tested on a bicycle ergometer and a motor-driven treadmill, after which they were randomly assigned to two different training groups. One group trained by pedaling a stationary bicycle, and the other group by running on the treadmill. At the end of 6 weeks of training, each group was retested on both the bicycle and the treadmill. Interestingly, even though both training procedures involved leg work, the bicycle group improved only when tested on the bicycle ergometer, but the treadmill group improved on both the bicycle and the treadmill. From these data, it appears that cycling is a more specific exercise, while running appears to be a more general conditioner. Other experiments comparing arm work and leg work have produced similar results: improvement seems to be restricted to the location of the working muscles [18]. Obviously, however, local muscle groups do not improve appreciably without some adaptation of the central circulation to training. Consequently, when constructing training programs, one must be careful to select stimuli that elicit central circulatory adaptation as well as peripheral adaptation in those muscles doing the work.

Second, the principle of overload (see Chapter 3) must be reemphasized: without a *stressor* (exercise) greater than that which is habitually encountered, no improvement will occur. The greater the overload, within certain limits, the greater the stimulus imposed.

Third, training must occur regularly at an intensity greater than a minimum threshold, or adaptation will not occur. The amount of the benefit, to a point, is roughly proportional to the amount of work accomplished.

Fourth, once the desired state of fitness is achieved, continued maintenance is necessary or the training effect will be lost. The rate of decline varies among individuals but appears to be influenced by a number of factors including heredity; the level, length, and type of prior training; and posttraining life-style. In general, physical fitness is lost more rapidly than it is achieved. A reasonable level of fitness can be maintained through biweekly or triweekly maintenance workouts.

TRAINING FOR CIRCULORESPIRATORY ENDURANCE

Circulorespiratory (CR) endurance (also called *aerobic power*) indicates a high state of efficiency of the circulatory and respiratory systems in supplying oxygen to the working tissue. Of all the benefits one might receive from physical training, increased CR endurance is perhaps the most important. There are a multitude of training styles for CR improvement. Two of the most popular are described here.

Continuous Exercise

It has been clearly established that running or jogging long, slow distances (LSD) is an excellent method of improving CR endurance. (**Jogging** is defined as a slow running pace of about 8 to 12 min/mile). Depending on the individual's training objective, appropriate distances range from 2 to 6 miles at an intensity of between 6 and 15 min/mile. Whatever the distance, the pace must be severe enough to elicit a heart rate of at least 60% of the maximum heart rate range, as was described in Chapter 3. Generally, this works out to be about 150 beats per minute for most people 18 to 25 years old.

The importance of the distance-intensity relationship can be clearly seen in the results of a study conducted by the authors, using 20 college-age women enrolled in a foundations class [4]. They ran

1.3 miles a day in symmetrically spaced triweekly sessions for 10 weeks. Although the women were aware of the intensity levels necessary to elicit a training response, they were not forced to work at any particular intensity; only the distance was required. A comparison of their treadmill performances before and after the training period revealed no changes in maximum oxygen uptake, heart rate response to a given submaximum work load, or maximum heart rate. It was concluded that distance alone in the absence of some minimum level of intensity does not guarantee improvements in CR endurance.

Interval Training

In the last decade, a style called **interval training** has been well received as an outstanding method of developing aerobic power. In contrast to the LSD regimen, interval training is discontinuous. A typical interval workout consists of several (three to seven) work periods that are relatively short (usually 3 to 5 minutes each) and very strenuous (approximately 75% to 90% of maximum capacity). These are interspaced by rest periods during which the subject walks or jogs while partially recovering for the next work period. The length of the recovery period may be based on a previously set **work-relief ratio** of 1:1 or 1:2, or it may be judged sufficient when the heart rate has returned to 120 beats per minute as determined by palpation of the carotid artery.

Interval-style training appears to have several advantages over continuous work.

1. The intensity of the work can be greater because the work periods are relatively short.
2. The total amount of work accomplished within a given time can be greater.
3. More work can be accomplished with less discomfort.
4. The flexibility of the program helps reduce the boredom of prolonged continuous exercise.
5. The methods available for increasing the work load are more flexible.

The important considerations in the construction of an interval program are:

1. The length of the work period. At least 3 to 5 minutes are required if aerobic power is the objective.
2. The length of the rest period. Acceptable ratios of work to relief are 1:1 or 1:2.

3. The intensity of the work. In most cases, 75% to 90% of maximum capacity is recommended.
4. The number of work periods.

As the individual adapts physiologically to the training stimulus, the work load can be increased by:

1. An increase in the length of the work period
2. A decrease in the length of the rest period
3. An increase in the intensity of the work period
4. An increase in the number of work periods
5. Any combination of the above

Apparently, not all types of exercise are equally effective in improving aerobic power. For example, Fox et al. [26] reported post-training increases in maximum oxygen uptake when several short sprints served as the training stimulus. The sprinting periods (15 to 30 seconds each) were interspaced with rest periods in the work-relief ratio of 1:3. Using 10 subjects in a similar program, the authors have been unable to replicate these results [5]. In another study, Allen et al. [3] used triweekly sessions of circuit weight training to condition 33 college freshmen. During each 27-minute workout, 30-second work bouts were alternated with 60-second rest periods (work-relief ratio of 1:2). Even though heart rates during the entire 27-minute workout far exceeded the generally accepted threshold for the production of cardiovascular adaptation, no *hemodynamic* improvement was found. From these results it must be concluded that high heart rates alone do not stimulate training benefits but that the type of exercise is important.

The appropriateness of using very short work intervals for development of aerobic power remains questionable. Reports of increasing aerobic power by means of work periods of less than 2 minutes should be accepted with reservations until a greater body of data supporting these claims can be assembled.

Suitable Activities

Several popular activities can improve circulorespiratory fitness. To qualify, three criteria must be met. First, the activity must be primarily aerobic. This means that the CR system is capable of supplying most of the oxygen required by the working muscles during the activity. Second, the level of the work (training stimulus) must be great enough to tax the oxygen transport system. Third, the time spent in the activity must be long enough to engage the aerobic metabolism as the primary pathway for energy production.

Running is probably the most popular activity for developing CR fitness. It is natural and no special facilities or expensive equipment are necessary. There are some tips that the beginning runner would be wise to take advantage of. First, careful selection of running shoes is important for those who plan to run more than a mile or two several times a week. Second, proper warm-up and careful attention to stretching and flexibility exercises are important for the prevention of injury. Third, attention to proper clothing for various environmental conditions increases comfort and safety. Finally, slow progression in increasing distance and pace coupled with "listening to one's body" makes the running experience more rewarding and enjoyable.

Bicycling is also an excellent conditioner. Although the equipment required is more expensive than equipment for running, the physiological benefits are similar. In addition, cycling can be great family or group fun and can provide an active way to cover greater geographical distances than running. This activity is also recommended for individuals whose bodies do not respond favorably to weight-bearing exercise.

For those who like to confine their activity to smaller geographic limits, swimming, rope skipping [29, 55], and aerobic dance offer benefits similar to those of running and cycling. For additional examples as well as to determine the potential of an activity as a training stimulus, consult Table 6-10. Keep in mind that the values for Caloric costs vary as the intensity with which the activity is pursued increases or decreases.

HEMODYNAMIC RESPONSES
TO ENDURANCE TRAINING

The training programs previously described in this chapter elicit responses that are specific to the frequency, intensity, duration, and type of exercise engaged in. Furthermore, the changes of adaptation might differ with respect to the physiologic states—rest, submaximum work, and maximum work. The consensus of recent research appears to support the posttraining changes presented in Tables 4-1 and 4-2 and in Figure 4-1.

TABLE 4-1
HEMODYNAMIC CHANGES AT REST AND DURING SUBMAXIMUM
AND MAXIMUM WORK AFTER SEVERAL WEEKS OF
CIRCULORESPIRATORY ENDURANCE TRAINING

Parameter	At Rest	During Submaximum Work	During Maximum Work
Heart rate	Decrease	Decrease	No change; slight decrease
Stroke volume	Increase	Increase	Increase
Cardiac output	No change; decrease	No change; decrease*	Increase
Peripheral blood flow	Decrease	Decrease	Increase
Systolic blood pressure	Decrease; no change	Decrease; no change	Decrease; no change
Diastolic blood pressure	Decrease; no change	Decrease; no change	Decrease; no change
Oxygen extraction (ml O_2 per 100 ml blood)	No change; increase	No change; increase	Increase
Oxygen uptake (liters/min)	No change	No change decrease*	Increase

*Slight decrease is due to increased mechanical efficiency.

TABLE 4-2
PHYSIOLOGIC ADAPTATION OF VARIOUS PARAMETERS
TO SEVERAL WEEKS OF CIRCULORESPIRATORY
ENDURANCE TRAINING

Parameter	Direction of Change
Fibrinolysis	Increase; no change
Hemoglobin (total)	Increase
Metabolic enzymes (aerobic)	Increase
Muscle capillarization	No change; increase
Myocardial weight	Increase
Percentage of body fat	Decrease
Red blood cells per mm^3	No change; decrease*
Serum cholesterol	No change
HDL-cholesterol	Increase
LDL-cholesterol	Decrease
Serum triglycerides	Decrease
Total blood volume	Increase

*Marathon training.

TRAINING FOR STRENGTH

For many years, the main physiologic benefit ascribed to weight training has been in the development of muscular strength. DeLorme [20] wrote that weight-training methods can be clearly divided into two types: a high-resistance, low-repetition program for strength development, and a low-resistance, high-repetition program for improvement of muscular endurance. He further suggested that either type is incapable of producing the results obtained by the other.

DeLorme's technique of *progressive resistive exercise*, generally accepted as the standard of weight training during the late 1940s, called for 7 to 10 bouts (**sets**) of repetitive exercise, each set consisting of 10 to 12 repetitions. His patients tried to increase the number of repetitions (**repetition max**, or **RM**) they could execute daily. At the end of each week, a new maximum resistance that could be

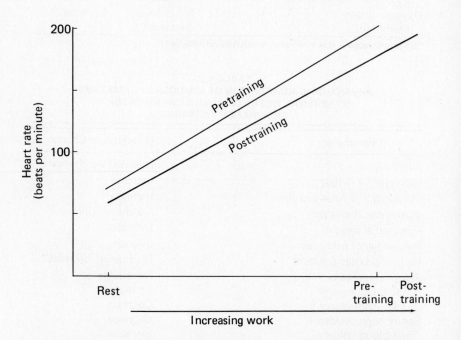

Figure 4-1. Heart rate response to given work loads before and after several weeks of endurance training.

handled through 10 repetitions (10 RM) was determined. The result was constant overload during the work period.

DeLorme and Watkins [21] later modified DeLorme's original statement on the necessary intensity and duration of the work bout; they recommended that patients (1) begin with only 50% of maximum contraction, to be increased to 100% at least once during the workout, and (2) reduce the seven to ten sets to two or three. This procedure was questioned by Zinovieff [58], who advocated reversing the order in which resistance is applied, so that the heaviest loads would be encountered first and reduced systematically thereafter to keep pace with fatigue.

Since the time of these early conceptions of technique, weight training has been studied extensively by several investigators. Differences of opinion based on practical experience as well as on the results of experimental research abound. Berger [10, 11, 12, 13] experimented with different combinations of repetitions and sets, attempting to identify the "best" method for developing strength. His findings supported the concept of high-resistance, low-repetition exercise recommended earlier by DeLorme. Furthermore, he concluded that a three-set, 6-RM regimen provided the best results. Workouts using heavier loads for fewer than 2 RM or lighter loads for more than 10 RM were not satisfactory alternatives to the three-set, 6-RM combination.

More recently, however, Stone et al. [52] have reported a method for developing strength which integrates the traditional approach with techniques employed by the very successful Eastern European strength coaches as well as by many body builders.

It is generally accepted that hypertrophied muscle has a higher potential for strength gain than nonhypertrophied muscle. According to Stone et al., hypertrophy is best achieved using three to five sets of relatively high-volume, low-resistance exercise (8 to 20 RM). Once the hypertrophy is achieved, three to five sets of 2 to 6 RM should be employed to produce the desired strength. In a study comparing this method with the traditional three-set, 6-RM method, these researchers reported the newer model to be superior to the more classical method for developing strength. Furthermore, the time required for a given amount of improvement with the newer model was reduced [52].

Isotonic Contraction

The strength programs mentioned above all make use of iso-tonic, also called dynamic or moving, contraction. An isotonic con-traction occurs when a muscle shortens and allows a joint to move through its complete range of motion. This occurs in natural move-ments such as walking and running. It also occurs in strength train-ing when conventional weights, or weight-training machines such as Universal and Nautilus, are employed.

Isometric Contraction

A second type of contraction used to overload muscles is isomet-ric. During isometric contraction, no shortening takes place—only straining against the resistance. Since the work of Hettinger and Muller [32] was first reported, it has been investigated extensively. Although not without opposition, some research supports isometrics as a useful method for developing muscular strength [10, 13, 27, 38, 40].

Originally, Hettinger and Muller reported that a single daily *static contraction* exceeding one-third of the maximum strength of a muscle and held for a short period was able to produce the maxi-mum rate of strength increase, whereas weekly contractions reduced the rate of gain by one-third [41]. The reported rapid increases in strength, with a minimum amount of time involved and with no equipment necessary, have made isometrics attractive. However, of several attempts [16, 30] to reproduce Hettinger and Muller's original findings, only one [44] was successful. Because strength appears to increase significantly only at the angle of the contraction, the authors do not consider isometric exercise programs to be effective in the development of strength for activities requiring dynamic contractions. In addition, reports of hypertensive blood-pressure response during heavy isometric work [23] and increased resting diastolic blood pressure after an isometric training regimen appear to contraindicate extensive use of isometrics, especially by those with a compromised heart or impaired arterial walls.

Perhaps the most valuable use of isometric contraction is by people who have sedentary jobs. Daily isometric exercise can be performed whether seated or standing and without attracting atten-tion. Moderate intensity contractions will serve to maintain muscle tone.

Isokinetic Contraction

A third and relatively new type of strength training is isokinetic exercise. *Isokinetic contraction*, unlike isotonic and isometric contraction, guarantees maximum resistance to movement and a constant rate of movement, regardless of the changes in force that take place as leverage and mechanical advantage change. It is well known that, after the initial force is applied during many lifts with conventional weights, the ballistic effect reduces the muscle force necessary to complete the movement. At the end of most conventional lifts, *eccentric contraction* must be used to brake the inertia and return the weight to the prelift position.

Many advocate the eccentric portion as a valuable part of strength development. Isokinetic exercise, with the help of specially designed devices, eliminates the eccentric portion of the movement and provides for a constant resistance, regardless of changes in the force generated by the contracting muscle. This means that the muscle encounters maximum resistance throughout its range of motion. Although several studies support isokinetics as more effective than isotonics or isometrics in strength improvement [33, 39, 46, 54], it could be argued that the elimination of eccentric contraction by isokinetics encourages an imbalance in opposing muscle groups and reduced coordination.

Steps in Developing a Strength Training Regimen

TRADITIONAL APPROACH

The program that follows is a "cookbook" approach to the formulation of one's own high-resistance, low-repetition program for strength development.

1. The individual must identify the muscle groups in which an increase in strength is desired.
2. Appropriate lifts to stimulate those muscles are selected.
3. The order of lifts is arranged in such a manner that the same muscle groups are not used consecutively.
4. For each lift, the maximum amount of weight that can be moved for a set of five repetitions is determined. This amount becomes the 5 RM.
5. The training regimen consists of three sets for each lift. Beginning with the 5 RM, the individual tries to work up to a maximum of eight repetitions for each lift during each of the first two sets.

6. When eight repetitions can be accomplished in each of the first two sets and exceeded in the third set, the resistance should be increased (at the beginning of the next training session) for that particular exercise until a new 5 RM (step 3) is established.
7. Lifting should occur triweekly on nonconsecutive days.

In the authors' laboratory 33 students using this program had an average gain in strength of 39% over a 12-week training period. The least improvement of the six muscle groups employed was 26%. The greatest amount of improvement, in the leg press, was 71% [3].

ANOTHER APPROACH

The program that follows is a straightforward approach for increasing strength at an optimum rate. It was constructed from a model developed by Dr. Michael Stone at the National Strength Research Center of Auburn University. Initially, a high-volume, low-intensity regimen is followed to produce muscular hypertrophy. Finally, a low-volume, high-intensity program is employed to increase strength in the hypertrophied muscle. Strength gains in a group using this model are reported to be significantly higher than in a group using the three-set, 6-RM program after 6 weeks of training [52]. The following nine steps should be helpful in personalizing this model:

1. Identify muscle groups to be strengthened.
2. Determine the kinds of lifts to be used.
3. Determine the 10 RM.
4. For 3 weeks employ three to five sets at 10 RM, 3 or 4 days a week.
5. For 4 weeks employ three sets at 5 RM, 3 or 4 days a week.
6. For 4 weeks employ three sets at 2 to 3 RM, 3 or 4 days a week.
7. Convert to a maintenance regimen or a program of active rest (training at a recreational level using low volume and low intensity).
8. Repeat the cycle.

RESPONSES TO STRENGTH TRAINING

The hemodynamic improvements that occur after several weeks of endurance training are not observed after strength training of equal duration. However, certain *histological* and biochemical changes are observed in the trained muscles.

1. Muscle fibers increase in size. There are also some reports of increase in the numbers of muscle fibers, but the evidence is not

convincing. At any rate, this is secondary in importance to individual fiber hypertrophy.
2. Contractile force (strength) increases.
3. Hypertrophy of connecting tendons, ligaments, and supporting bony structures takes place.
4. Articular cartilages become thicker and more compressible.
5. Oxidative enzyme concentration decreases.
6. Mitochondrial volume density decreases [36].

CIRCUIT TRAINING

Circuit training was introduced by Adamson [2] in the late 1950s. This method can be used to improve general body condition, or it can be combined with resistive exercises in a program of circuit weight training for the development of strength or muscular endurance.

The classic circuit program consists of 9 to 12 exercise stations arranged in a circuit. After choosing the amount of work to be performed at each station, the subject is timed during three laps around the circuit (with no rest between exercises or laps). The time recorded is reduced by one-third; the resulting figure is the target time. When the subject successfully completes the three laps within the target time, the amount of work at each station is increased, a new target time is established, and the training resumes.

MUSCLE SORENESS

Engagement in activities different from those to which one is usually accustomed often produces muscle soreness. This is normal and is observed after both strength work and endurance work. In some cases, pain has been reported to occur during the latter stages of high-intensity exercise. More often, it occurs as many as 24 to 48 hours after the activity. This kind of soreness, which appears several hours after the exercise, causes the most discomfort because it usually persists for several days.

The pain that accompanies heavy exercise most likely results from the accumulation of metabolic waste products such as *lactic acid.* This pain is transitory and usually subsides shortly after the intensity of the exercise is reduced. Recovery appears to be enhanced by continued, very mild movement. This encourages the removal of metabolic wastes from the affected muscles because it allows circulation to continue at a relatively higher level than what would be experienced if the exercise were stopped abruptly.

The soreness that occurs 24 to 48 hours after a heavy work bout and persists for several days is less well understood. At least three theories have been advanced to explain it. Hough [34] has hypothesized that the pain results from structural damage. DeVries [22] has proposed that the soreness results from spasms of localized motor units in the affected muscles. Assmussen [8] and Komi and Buskirk [35] have suggested that overstretching the muscle's elastic components during the eccentric phase of contraction produces the delayed pain.

In a study by Abraham [1], the validity of each theory was tested experimentally. He reported that the evidence did not appear to support either the spasm or the muscle-damage theory, and that the 24- to 48-hour delay can most likely be attributed to alterations in the muscle connective tissue (elastic components). However, the soreness was found to be present in muscles that performed concentric contractions as well as in those that performed eccentric ones.

Recovery from this type of soreness can be enhanced by warm compresses or warm baths, accompanied by light exercise to help prevent adhesions during the healing process.

EXERCISE INJURY

All who exercise should be aware that the benefits to be gained are not without concomitant risk of injury. In healthy individuals, exercise can induce injuries that range from minor aggravations to those so painful as to require complete immobilization during recovery. For others, such as postcoronary patients, persons in the CHD high risk category, and those with certain congenital abnormalities, some forms and levels of exercise can be hazardous—even life threatening. These people should exercise only under close medical supervision.

Each sports/recreational activity has its own category of injuries that are peculiar to its demands. Although complete categorization and coverage are beyond the scope of this book, a few of the injuries most common to runners and bicyclists will be described because these activities are probably the most popular forms of exercise at the present time.

Runner's Knee (Chondromalacia Patella)

Runner's knee is characterized by pain in the area of the knee. It has been described as the most frequent overuse injury in sports. According to Dr. George Sheehan [49], four factors can act singly or in combination to produce an erosion of the cartilage covering the underside of the kneecap. The factors are structural instability of the foot, postural instability, leg-length discrepancy, and environmental stresses such as improper shoes or running on slanting surfaces. A weak quadraceps muscle (anterior thigh) has also been implicated.

To alleviate the condition, usually the foot must be treated rather than the knee. Foot supports called orthotics are placed in the shoes to assure balanced bone structure in the foot and ankle. Flexibility exercises are prescribed to stretch the shortened hamstring muscles. Lifts are used to equalize leg length. And properly constructed training shoes with adequate foot cushion are recommended.

Achilles Tendinitis

Achilles tendinitis is an inflammation of the heel cord (Achilles tendon) common in those who participate in running sports. It is most often the result of shortened calf muscles or of an abnormally formed foot that puts stress on the cord. It can be prevented by using stretching exercises to lengthen the calf and by inserting a wedge to elevate the heel adequately.

Use of ice on the area, heel lift orthotics, flexibility exercises, and the avoidance of hill and speed running are recommended during the treatment and recovery period [49, 51].

Shinsplints

Shinsplints is a general term for pain over the anterior lower leg. It could result from a stress fracture of the lower leg bone (tibia), or ischemia of the posterior leg compartment, or even soft-tissue injury and inflammation [9]. Overuse of the anterior compartment muscles, strength and flexibility imbalance of the lower leg muscles, a weak and pronated foot, and improper shoes are factors often cited as contributing to the development of this disorder.

Treatment employs ice on the painful area, elevation, and rest, plus correcting the factors creating the problem.

Stress Fractures

Stress fractures are overuse injuries resulting from a series of submaximum stresses, any one of which is unlikely to cause a fracture. They are commonly seen in the long bones of the feet (metatarsals) and the bones of the lower leg (tibia and fibula) of middle- and long-distance runners [48].

The chief symptom is diffuse pain that later localizes. This disorder is difficult to diagnose because these fractures may not be visible in an X-ray for several days [43].

Colored Urine (Pigmenturia)

In some long-distance runners, the release of hemoglobin due to red blood cell destruction (hemoglobinuria) or of myoglobin during muscle damage (myoglobinuria) can result in pigmented urine during the first few hours after completing a run [19]. This type of pigmenturia is not dangerous nor is it an indication of a pathological condition. With adequate fluid replacement, the disorder usually corrects itself in a few hours.

Another form of pigmenturia results from red blood cells in the urine (hematuria) owing to bladder or urethra damage from repeated pounding of the bladder walls during long-distance running (usually 10,000 meters or longer). This form usually corrects itself also within 24 to 48 hours. In any of these pigmenturias, dark urine beyond 48 hours warrants prompt medical evaluation.

Of concern should be the underlying cause. Some doctors feel that the degree of exertion by the average jogger is not likely to produce hematuria from bladder trauma, and that all such first events should be clinically evaluated in light of the possibility of kidney or bladder tumors, cysts, stones, or other urinary disorders [14, 17]. Others contend that first episodes which correct themselves are not usually dangerous and do not warrant the cost and inconvenience of complete urinary tract evaluation [50].

It has been suggested that hematuria from bladder trauma might be prevented if a critical volume of urine remains in the bladder to cushion the shock during exercise [15]. To accomplish this, the runner refrains from complete bladder evacuation prior to running. Another technique involves full hydration prior to and during exercise.

Blisters and Stone Bruises

A blister is an escape of tissue fluid beneath the skin's surface caused by friction. Although they are debilitating to a runner, blisters usually heal relatively quickly compared to other exercise-induced injuries. Recovery time is prolonged, however, if improper care allows them to become infected.

Selection of properly fitting footwear, lubricating the areas of friction, and sensible care of the feet can prevent most blisters. When they do occur, the affected area should be cleansed with an antiseptic. The blister should then be lanced with a sterile needle at several points along its circumference and forcibly drained. The dead skin layer should be allowed to remain in place for protection. It is helpful to surround the affected area with a thin felt or sponge doughnut to relieve pressure and eliminate friction until the area ceases to be tender.

Stone bruises of the heel surface or the ball of the foot are most often caused by running with inadequate foot cushion on rocky surfaces. The use of a sponge doughnut is about the only treatment unless one chooses to stay off the injured foot until it has healed.

Many of the other overuse injuries incurred by runners could be prevented by adequate attention to strengthening anterior surface muscles and stretching posterior surface muscles. The low back problems frequently experienced result from muscle strength imbalances in the abdomen and lower spine area. A regular flexibility regimen using bent-knee situps to strengthen abdominal muscles while at the same time increasing lower back flexibility has proven helpful.

Bicycling Injury

Poor riding position while bicycling encourages problems with the back, neck, and hands. The common cause is a combination of maladjustments that place the trunk too far forward. To see ahead, the neck must be hyperextended. Over a long ride the required activity of the neck muscles may lead to severe localized neck pain or headache.

To support the trunk against gravity, either the muscles of the lower back must work continuously or the hands and arms must support the weight of the trunk. Continuous sharing of the load by the back muscles often leads to low back pain. Too much weight on the hands for extended periods can lead to serious neurological damage to the hand.

During the exaggerated trunk-forward position, typical hand placement on the handlebar subjects the ulnar nerve to severe punishment. In the hand, this nerve runs along the palmar surface on the side of the ring finger. Nerve fiber compression resulting from prolonged support of the trunk weight coupled with the periodic shocks transmitted from the riding surface through the frame results in a loss of the nerve's ability to transmit impulses. The symptoms of this injury are loss of sensation or tingling in the ring and little finger on either or both hands and weakness in one or both hands; both symptoms may occur simultaneously. Compression neuropathy can result in irreversible damage to the ulnar nerve and permanent paralysis to the hand.

This disorder can be prevented by improved riding position, frequent change in hand position on the handlebar, and padding the handlebar or wearing padded gloves [24].

Dehydration and Heat Illness

All exercisers should appreciate the necessity of water and electrolyte replacement when working in the heat. Weighing in before and after working out can serve as a guide to the amount of water that needs to be replaced. If a preworkout weight is 2% or more under the preworkout weight of the previous day, fluid replacement probably has been inadequate. Generally, for each pound of weight lost because of sweating, 1 pint of supplemental water is required.

Although less critical than fluid replacement, electrolyte replacement is very important for maintenance of health. After acclimatization to exercising in the heat has occurred, dietary intake of sodium and potassium is usually sufficient to maintain safe levels except in those who sweat profusely. Even in these cases, supplemental salt is not required until more than 6 pounds have been lost during one workout. The resulting deficit is then best handled by slightly increasing the amount of salt used at the table. Salt tablets are not recommended, because of the digestive disturbances so often related to their ingestion. A word of caution: if salt tablets are used, copious amounts of water are required (at least 1 pint per 7-grain tablet) or severe medical consequences might result [37].

Inadequate water and electrolyte replacement and disregard of safe practices when working in the heat can lead to heat cramps, heat fatigue, and heatstroke. Symptoms of heat cramps and heat fatigue are usually transitory and disappear after a few hours of rest in a cooler environment and ingestion of fluids. Heatstroke, on the other hand, is life threatening, and most persons do not recover without prompt medical attention. Even then, permanent damage to the thermal regulatory mechanism usually results.

The best way to prevent heatstroke and other forms of heat illness is through adequate water and electrolyte replacement and the use of good judgment when working in the heat. The American College of Sports Medicine's position statement on such matters as fluid replacement while exercising is very helpful [7].

WOMEN AND TRAINING

In recent years women have become more involved in physical activity and athletic competition. In most cases, the female response to physical training is identical to the male response. There are, however, a few special problems common to women.

Iron Depletion

After the onset of the menstrual cycle, some women become more susceptible to iron-related blood disorders because they lose iron during menstruation. Some studies have reported that prolonged, regular exercise (training) tends to aggravate this problem by reducing the body's store of iron. Although the literature is not in complete agreement [42, 57], sufficient evidence exists to suggest that women engaged in prolonged heavy training should have their serum iron levels monitored to determine whether they need supplemental iron.

Menstrual Cycle and Exercise

The regularity of the menstrual period varies widely among healthy women, and so does the degree of associated discomfort. The best advice regarding exercise during menstruation appears to be "listen to your body." If it says no, then exercise should be postponed, or at least curtailed, until normal vigor returns. Although exercising during menses is not harmful, heavy work may not be well tolerated. In the authors' laboratory two women experienced very uncomfortable responses to maximum treadmill testing during their menstrual periods.

A growing body of evidence suggests that severe, prolonged training, such as long-distance running, is associated with the cessation of menstrual periods (amenorrhea) and the absence of ovulation [6, 25, 53]. Whether this departure from normal reproductive function results directly from exercise or indirectly from the dramatic reduction of body fat typical of long-distance runners is not clear. It is known that severe reduction of body fat in females inhibits the production of hormones that regulate the menstrual cycle. This appears to be transitory, however, and menstrual function returns to normal when training ceases or becomes less intense. Although heavy exercise is not recommended as a safe method of birth control, women trying to become pregnant should be aware that hard training may reduce fertility.

Breast Soreness

Breast soreness is a frequent complaint of many women who exercise regularly. Haycock and Gillette [31] reported that 72% of the female athletes they questioned experienced sore or tender breasts after exercise, most commonly after running. Although the reason for this soreness is not known, most theories attribute it to the stress produced on the underlying muscle and connective tissue by the horizontal and vertical motion of the breast during vigorous body movement.

Apparently, factors other than breast size (mass) contribute to the discomfort. In a study designed to investigate breast soreness, Gehlsen and Albohm [28] studied 20 female athletes, 10 of whom had felt breast discomfort and 10 of whom had never felt breast discomfort. The bra cup sizes of the women in the discomfort group were 50% B, 20% C, and 30% D. The cup sizes of those who felt no discomfort were 90% B and 10% D. Biomechanical analysis of breast motion during running showed that the two groups differed significantly only in the product of breast mass and velocity of movement. It was concluded that the breast mass, acting in conjunction with the velocity of breast movement, may be related to discomfort while jogging.

If the breasts of exercising women are not properly supported, damage to underlying muscle and connective tissue may result. This could lead to premature breast sag. If this is true, an exercise bra would be a wise investment. The desirable qualities of such a bra, suggested by finalists in a recent women's marathon, are firm lateral support; sufficient total support; no lace, padding, or underwires; an all-elastic back; and a wide variety of sizes. An interesting study of the effectiveness of sports bras showed that breast motion can be controlled by a properly constructed bra [28, 47]. Therefore, women who wear a B or larger cup should consider wearing a sports bra when exercising.

REFERENCES

1. Abraham, W. M. Factors in delayed muscle soreness. *Medicine and Science in Sports* 9 (1):11–20, 1977.
2. Adamson, G. T. Circuit training. *Ergonomics* 2:183–186, 1959.
3. Allen, T. E.; Byrd, R. J.; and Smith, D. P. Hemodynamic consequences of circuit weight training. *Research Quarterly* 47:299–305, 1976.
4. Allen, T. E., and Miller, D. K. The effects of 10 weeks of running at volitional intensity on the cardiovascular systems of college women. *Journal of Physical Education and Recreation* 49 (6):75–76, 1978.
5. ———. Sprint training for aerobic power. Unpublished report. Wilmington: University of North Carolina.
6. American College of Sports Medicine. Opinion statement: Participation of the female athlete in long-distance running. *Medicine and Science in Sports* 11 (4):IX, 1979.
7. American College of Sports Medicine. Position statement: Prevention of heat injuries during distance running. *Medicine and Science in Sports* 7 (1):VII, 1975.
8. Assmussen, E. Observations on experimental muscle soreness. *Acta Rheumatologica Scandinavica* 1:109–116, 1956.
9. Benas, D., and Jokl, P. Shin splints. *American Corrective Therapy Journal* 32 (2):53–57, 1978.
10. Berger, R. A. Comparison of static and dynamic strength increases. *Research Quarterly* 33:329–333, 1962.
11. ———. Effect of varied weight training programs on strength. *Research Quarterly* 33:168–181, 1962.
12. ———. Optimum repetitions for the development of strength. *Research Quarterly* 33:334–338, 1962.
13. ———. Comparison between static training and various dynamic training programs. *Research Quarterly* 34:131–135, 1963.
14. Blacklock, N. J. Bladder trauma from jogging. *American Heart Journal* 99 (6):813–814, 1980.
15. ———. Bladder trauma in the long-distance runner. *American Journal of Sports Medicine* 7 (4):239–241, 1979.
16. Bonde-Petersen, F. Muscle training by static, concentric, and eccentric contractions. *Acta Physiologica Scandinavica* 48:406–416, 1960.
17. *British Medical Journal*. The haematuria of the long-distance runner. 6183 (2):159, 1979.
18. Clausen, J. P.; Trap-Jensen, J.; and Lassen, N. A. The effects of training on the heart rate during arm and leg exercise. *Scandinavian Journal of Clinical and Laboratory Investigation* 26:295–301, 1970.
19. Daniels, J.; Fitts, R.; and Sheehan, G. *Conditioning for distance running*. New York: John Wiley and Sons, 1978.
20. DeLorme, T. L. Restoration of muscle power by heavy resistance exercise. *Archives of Physical Medicine* 27:645–667, 1945.
21. DeLorme, T. L., and Watkins, A. L. Techniques of progressive resistance exercise. *Archives of Physical Medicine* 29:263–273, 1948.
22. deVries, H. A. Quantitative electromyographic investigation of the spasm theory of muscle pain. *American Journal of Physical Medicine* 45:119–134, 1966.

23. Donald, K. W.; Lind, A. R.; McNicol, G. W.; Humphreys, P. W.; Taylor, S. H.; and Staunton, H. P. Cardiovascular responses to sustained (static) contractions. *Physiology of Muscular Exercise.* American Heart Association Monograph no. 15, 15–30, 1967.

24. Faria, I. E., and Cavanagh, P. R. *The physiology and biomechanics of cycling.* New York: John Wiley and Sons, 1978.

25. Feicht, C. B.; Johnson, T. S.; Martin, B. J.; Sparkes, K. E.; and Wagner, W. W. Secondary amenorrhoea in athletes. Letter to the editor, *Lancet* 2 (8100):1145–1146, 1978.

26. Fox, E. L.; Bartels, R. L.; Billings, C. E.; Matthews, D. K.; Batson, P.; and Webb, W. M. Intensity and distance of interval training programs and changes in aerobic power. *Medicine and Science in Sports* 5:18–22, 1973.

27. Gardner, G. W. Specificity of strength changes of the exercised and non-exercised limb following isometric training. *Research Quarterly* 34:529–537, 1963.

28. Gehlsen, G., and Albohm, M. Evaluation of sports bras. *The Physician and Sportsmedicine* 8 (10):89–97, 1980.

29. Getchel, B., and Cleary, P. The caloric cost of rope skipping and running. *The Physician and Sportsmedicine* 8 (2):56–60, 1980.

30. Hansen, J. W. The training effect of repeated isometric muscle contractions. *Internationale Zeitschrift fur Angewandte Physiologie* 18:474–477, 1961.

31. Haycock, C. E., and Gillette, J. Susceptibility of women athletes to injury. *Journal of the American Medical Association* 236:163–164, 1976.

32. Hettinger, T., and Muller, E. A. Muskelleistung and muskeltraining. *Arbeitsphysiologie* 15:111–126, 1953.

33. Hislop, H. J., and Perrine, J. J. The isokinetic concept of exercise. *Physical Therapy* 47 (2):114–117, 1967.

34. Hough, T. Ergographic studies in muscular soreness. *American Journal of Physiology* 7:76–92, 1902.

35. Komi, P. V., and Buskirk, E. R. The effect of eccentric and concentric muscle activity on tension and electrical activity of human muscles. *Ergonomics* 15:417–434, 1972.

36. MacDougall, J. D.; Sale, D. G.; Moroz, J. R.; Elder, G. C. B.; Sutton, J. R.; and Howard, H. Mitochondrial volume density in human skeletal muscle following heavy resistance training. *Medicine and Science in Sports* 11 (2):164–166, 1979.

37. Mathews, D. K., and Fox, E. L. *The physiological basis of physical education and athletics.* 2d ed. Philadelphia: W. B. Saunders Company, 1976.

38. Mathews, D. K., and Kruse, R. Effects of isometric and isotonic exercises on elbow flexor muscle groups. *Research Quarterly* 29:26–37, 1957.

39. Moffroid, M.; Whipple, R.; Hofkosh, J.; Lowman, E.; and Thistle, H. A study of isokinetic exercise. *Physical Therapy* 49 (7):735–747, 1965.

40. Morehouse, C. A. Development and maintenance of isometric strength of subjects with diverse initial strength. *Research Quarterly* 38:449–456, 1967.

41. Muller, E. A. Training muscle strength. *Ergonomics* 2:216–222, 1958.

42. Puhl, J. L., and Runyan, W. S. Hematological variations during aerobic training of college women. *Research Quarterly* 51 (3):533–541, 1980.
43. Quigley, T. B., ed. *1979 Yearbook of sports medicine.* Chicago: Year Book Medical Publishers, 1979.
44. Rarick, G. L., and Larsen, G. L. Observations on frequency and intensity of isometric muscular effort in developing static muscular strength in postpubescent males. *Research Quarterly* 29:333–341, 1958.
45. Roberts, J. A., and Alspaugh, J. W. Specificity of training effects resulting from treadmill running and bicycle ergometer riding. *Medicine and Science in Sports* 4:6–10, 1972.
46. Rosentswieg, J., and Hinson, M. M. Comparison of isometric, isotonic and isokinetic exercises by electromyography. *Archives of Physical Medicine and Rehabilitation* 53 (6):249–252, 1972.
47. Schuster, K. Equipment update: Jogging bras hit the streets. *The Physician and Sportsmedicine* 7 (4):125–128, 1979.
48. Scriber, K., and Burke, E. J., eds. *Relevant topics in athletic training.* Ithaca, N.Y.: Movement Publications, 1978.
49. Sheehan, G. *Medical advice for runners.* Mountain View, Calif.: World Publications, 1978.
50. Siegel, A. J.; Hennekens, C. H.; Solomon, H. S.; and Boeckel, B. V. Exercise related hematuria: Findings in a group of marathon runners. *Journal of the American Medical Association* 241 (4):391–392, 1979.
51. Smart, G. W.; Tauton, J. E.; and Clement, D. B. Achilles tendon disorders in runners—a review. *Medicine and Science in Sports and Exercise* 12 (4):231–243, 1980.
52. Stone, M. H.; O'Bryant, H.; and Garhammer, J. A hypothetical model for strength training. *Journal of Sports Medicine and Physical Fitness,* in press.
53. Strauss, R. H., ed. *Sports medicine and physiology.* Philadelphia: W. B. Saunders Company, 1979.
54. Thistle, H. G.; Hislop, H. J.; Moffroid, M.; and Lowman, E. W. Isokinetic contraction: new concept of resistive exercise. *Archives of Physical Medicine and Rehabilitation* 48 (6):279–282, 1967.
55. Town, G. P.; Sol, N.; and Sinning, W. E. The effect of rope skipping rate on energy expenditure of males and females. *Medicine and Science in Sports and Exercise* 12 (4):295–298, 1980.
56. Van Huss, W. D.; Niemeyer, R. K.; Olson, H. W.; and Friedrich, J. A. *Physical activity in modern living.* 2d ed. Englewood Cliffs, N.J.: Prentice-Hall, 1969.
57. Wirth, J. C.; Lohman, T. G.; Avallone, J. P.; Shire, T.; and Boileau, R. A. The effect of physical training on the serum iron levels of college-age women. *Medicine and Science in Sports* 10 (3):223–226, 1978.
58. Zinovieff, A. N. Heavy resistance exercises. *British Journal of Physical Medicine* 14:129–132, 1951.

KEY TERMS
Ballistic stretch (p. 69)
Flexibility (p. 68)
Static stretch (p. 69)
Stretch reflex (p. 69)

BEHAVIORAL OBJECTIVES
Upon completion of this chapter the student
should be able to:
1. Define the key terms listed above.
2. Describe six problems and disorders associated with inflexibility and four advantages of good flexibility.
3. Determine his or her neck, shoulder, chest, trunk, lower back, hips and hamstring muscles flexibility.
4. Design an individualized program to develop flexibility.
5. Develop flexibility in joints where there is inflexibility.

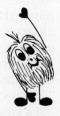

Flexibility is the ability of an individual to move the body joints through a maximum range of motion without undue strain. It is not a general factor but is specific to given joints and to particular sports or physical activities. It is more dependent on the soft tissues (ligaments, tendons, and muscles) of a joint than on the bony structure of the joint itself [2]. However, the bony structures of certain joints do place limitations on flexibility as illustrated by the extension of the elbow or the knee. Similarly, *hyperextension* of the spinal column is limited by the position and shape of the spinous processes, as bending or abduction is limited by the position and shape of the transverse processes.

Flexibility is also related to body size, sex, age, and activity. Any increase in body fat usually decreases flexibility. Females are generally more flexible than males of the same age. From birth to old age, there is a gradual decrease in flexibility as the soft tissues lose their extensibility [4]. This decrease is usually caused by failure to maintain an active program of movement through a complete range of motion.

Active individuals tend to be more flexible than inactive individuals, because flexibility is predominantly a function of habits of movement. The soft tissues or joints tend to shrink and thus lose extensibility when the muscles are maintained in a shortened position, as happens in sedentary individuals. Habitual postures and chronic heavy work through restricted ranges of motion also can lead to adaptive shortening of muscles. Physical activity with wide ranges of movement helps prevent this loss of extensibility. In summary, flexibility is related to habitual movement patterns for each individual and for each joint, and age and sex differences are secondary rather than innate [4].

EFFECTS OF INFLEXIBILITY

Flexibility is an important aspect of physical fitness, and the lack of it can create disorders or functional problems for many individuals. Anyone with a stiff spinal column is at a disadvantage in many physical activities and also fails to get full value from the shock-absorbing arrangement of the spine when walking, running, or jumping. Lack of flexibility in the back can also be responsible for bad posture, compression of peripheral nerves, painful menstruation, and other ailments [4]. Short muscles limit work efficiency. They become sore when they perform physical exertion, and, without a good range of movement, the individual is more likely to incur torn ligaments and muscles during activities. In summary, individuals with good flexibility have greater ease of movement, less stiffness of muscles, enhancement of skill, and less chance of injury during movement.

DEVELOPMENT OF FLEXIBILITY

It is impossible to state how much flexibility is desirable, but everyone should strive to prevent loss of flexibility during the aging process. It is accepted that, of the soft tissues, the muscles are most affected by stretching exercises and that both the **static stretch** (a holding position) and the **ballistic stretch** (a bouncing motion) are effective in the development of flexible joints. However, the use of a fast, forceful, bobbing type of stretching induces the **stretch reflex,** which could result in injury to muscle tissue. The amount and rate of the stretch reflex contraction vary directly in proportion to the amount and rate of the movement that causes the stretch. The faster and more forceful the stretch, the faster and more forceful the reflex contraction of the stretched muscle. Static stretching is recommended because it will not induce the stretch reflex. In addition, it poses less danger of exceeding the extensibility limits of the tissues involved, it requires less expenditure of energy, and it provides greater relief from muscle soreness [1].

Stretching should never proceed to the point of actual pain and subsequent soreness. There will usually be some discomfort, but any aftereffects that do occur should be carefully noted and given time to repair.

Little is known about the minimum requirement for the production of gains in flexibility, but experience has shown that improvement is most likely to result from *distributed practice* rather than from *massed practice* [2]. It is better to do sets of stretches for each specific flexibility throughout the day than to do all of them at once. Daily exercise, or at least five days per week, is also recommended. Once the desired flexibility has been attained, three days of exercise per week are probably adequate to maintain flexibility [2].

The most important specific flexibilities are probably neck and shoulder flexion, back extension, hip flexion, and posterior lower-leg extension (ankle flexion). Hip flexion is performed with the knees straight to stretch the hamstrings (posterior upper-leg muscles). Tight hamstrings cause an improper pelvic tilt, which is a potential contributor to lower back pain or problems [2].

GUIDELINES FOR DEVELOPMENT OF FLEXIBILITY

The following guidelines are recommended for flexibility programs [2].

1. Practice regularly. Flexibility exercises should be performed several times per day and at least five days per week.
2. Flexibility is highly specific to each joint and activity; therefore, flexibility exercises are highly specific.
3. Stretch gently and gradually to prevent soreness and damage to tissues.
4. The extent of stretching should be gradually and progressively enlarged with full extension, flexion, or both being placed on the joint.
5. Flexibility can accompany strength development if exercises are performed through the full range of joint movement.

MEASUREMENT OF FLEXIBILITY

It should be repeated that flexibility is not a general factor but is specific to each joint. No single test, therefore, can measure the flexibility of all the major joints of the body. In addition, there are two types of flexibility tests:

1. Relative flexibility tests are designed to be relative to the length or width of a specific body part. In these tests the movement and the length or width of an influencing body part are measured.
2. Absolute flexibility tests are designed to measure only the movement in relation to an absolute performance goal.

The following absolute flexibility tests provide an indication of flexibility in various parts of the body. (See Table 5-1 for desirable scores for these tests.)

The shoulder lift test (see Figure 5-1) measures flexibility of the shoulders and the shoulder girdle.

1. Lie prone on the floor. Touch the chin to the floor and extend the arms forward directly in front of the shoulders.
2. Hold a stick or ruler horizontally with both hands. Keep the elbows and wrists straight.
3. Raise the arms upward as far as possible with the chin still touching the floor. Measure the distance in inches from the bottom of the stick or ruler to the floor.

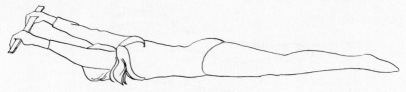

Figure 5-1. Shoulder lift test.

The trunk extension test (see Figure 5-2) measures flexibility of the trunk.

1. Lie prone on the floor with a partner holding the buttocks and legs down.
2. With fingers interlocked behind the neck, raise the chest and head off the floor as far as possible. Measure the distance in inches from the floor to the chin.

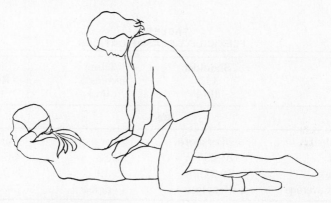

Figure 5-2. Trunk extension test.

The sit and reach test (see Figure 5-3) measures flexibility of the trunk and the hips.

1. Sit on the floor with the legs fully extended and the feet flat against a bench turned on its side.
2. While a partner holds the knees straight, bend forward and extend the arms and hands as far as possible.
3. Measure the distance from the fingertips to the edge of the bench. If the fingers do not reach the edge, the distance is expressed as a negative score, and if they reach beyond the edge, it is expressed as a positive score.

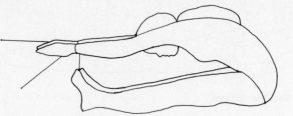

Figure 5-3. Sit and reach test.

TABLE 5-1
FLEXIBILITY CLASSIFICATIONS

	Shoulder Lift (in.)	Trunk Extension (in.)	Sit and Reach (in.)
Men			
Excellent	26 or more	23 or more	7 or more
Good	23-25	20-22	4-6
Average	20-22	18-19	1-3
Below average	19 or less	17 or less	0
Women			
Excellent	25 or more	20 or more	8 or more
Good	21-24	17-19	5-7
Average	18-20	15-16	2-4
Below average	17 or less	14 or less	0-1

SOURCES: C.B. Corbin, et al., *Concepts in physical education*, 2d ed. (Dubuque: William C. Brown, 1974); and R.V. Hockey, *Physical fitness—the pathway to healthful living*, 3rd ed. (St. Louis: C.V. Mosby, 1977).

The procedures shown in Figures 5-4 through 5-7 can also be performed to measure flexibility [3].

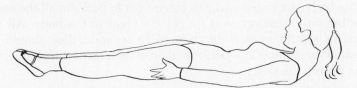

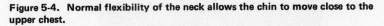

Figure 5-4. Normal flexibility of the neck allows the chin to move close to the upper chest.

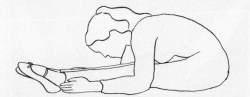

Figure 5-5. Normal flexibility of the hips and lower back allows flexion to about 135° in a young adult.

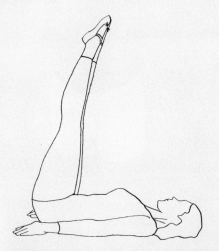

Figure 5-6. Normal flexibility of the hamstring muscle allows straight-leg lifting to 90° from a supine position.

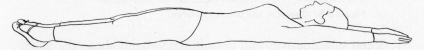

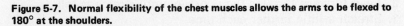

Figure 5-7. Normal flexibility of the chest muscles allows the arms to be flexed to 180° at the shoulders.

EXERCISES TO DEVELOP FLEXIBILITY

The following exercises are designed to develop flexibility throughout the body. An individual can choose not to perform all the exercises but only to select ones for certain areas of the body. All the
exercises should have a duration of 20 seconds; they should be
repeated three times and performed on at least three different occasions during the day.

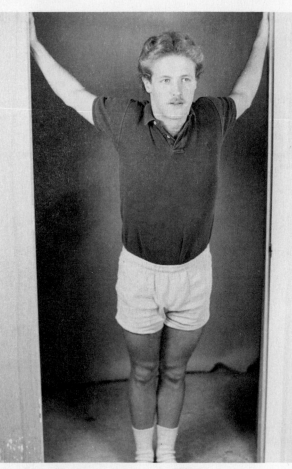

Figure 5-8. Shoulder and pectoral stretch.

1. Stand in a doorway and grasp the doorjamb above the head.
2. Lean forward through the doorway until stretch is felt.
3. Stretch a little farther each time.

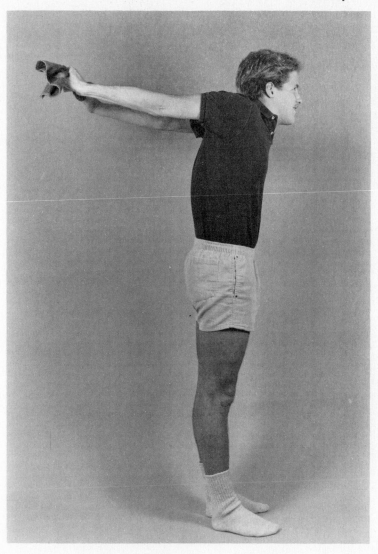

Figure 5-9. Shoulder and pectoral stretch.

1. Stand and hold a towel behind the hips, with the elbows straight and the palms toward the rear.
2. Lift the hands backward as high as possible.
3. Stretch a little farther each time. Do not bend forward.

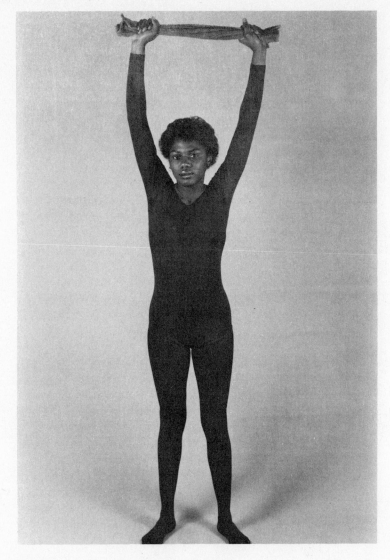

Figure 5-10. Shoulder and pectoral stretch.

1. Stand and hold a towel in front of the body, with the elbows straight and the palms down, about 18 in. apart.
2. Slowly lift the towel forward and overhead.

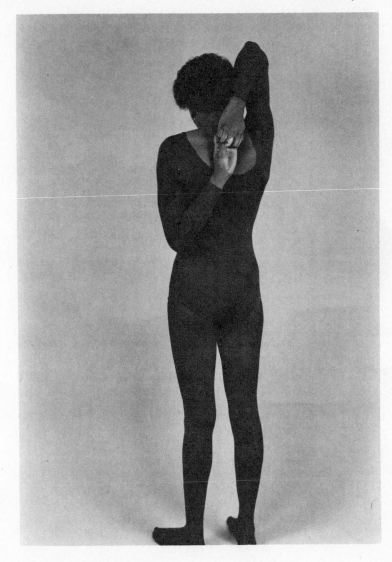

Figure 5-11. Shoulder stretch.

1. Bring the right hand over the right shoulder to the upper back.
2. Bring the left hand under the left shoulder to the upper back.
3. Hook the fingers of the two hands together and pull.

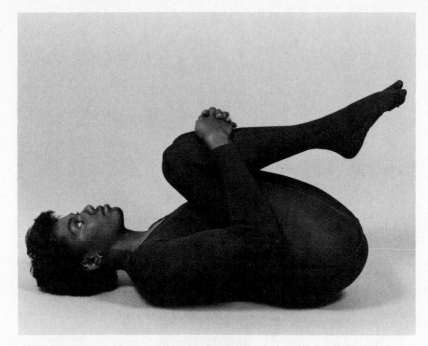

Figure 5-12. Back extensors stretch.

1. Lie supine with the knees flexed and the feet flat on the floor.
2. Pull in the stomach and bring both knees toward the center.
3. Grasp the knees and pull them toward the chest.

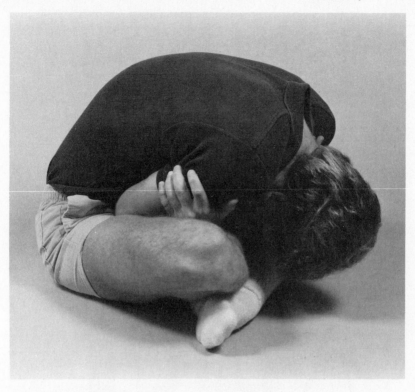

Figure 5-13.   Back extensors stretch.

1. Sit with the legs crossed and the arms folded across the chest.
2. Tuck the chin and curl forward. Try to touch the forehead to the knees.

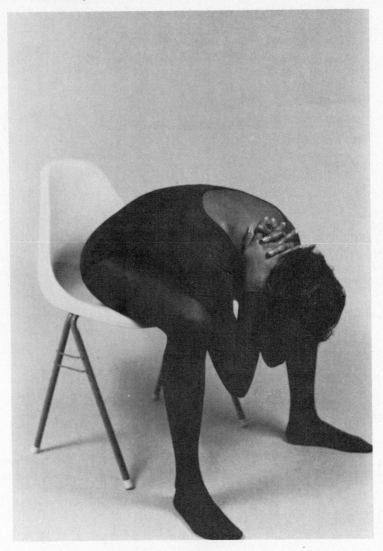

Figure 5-14. Back extensors stretch.

1. Sit in a chair with the feet about 24 inches apart.
2. Bend forward, with the arms and shoulders between the knees.
3. Attempt to touch the elbows to the floor.
4. Stretch until stretch discomfort is felt in the lower back.

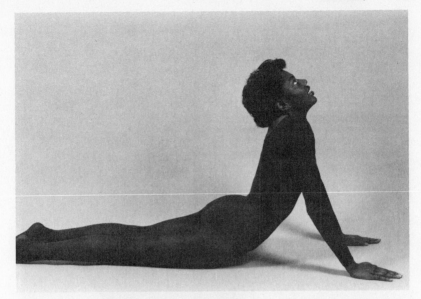

Figure 5-15. Upper trunk stretch.

1. Lie prone with the hands in the push-up position.
2. Extend the arms fully to raise the shoulders and upper back. Keep the pelvis and legs on the floor.

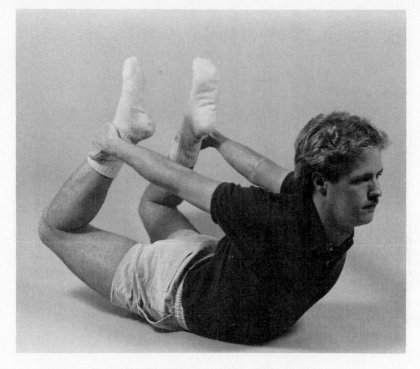

Figure 5-16. Lower trunk stretch.

1. Lie prone, bend the lower legs, and reach back and grasp the ankles.
2. Pull slowly and hold the head up.

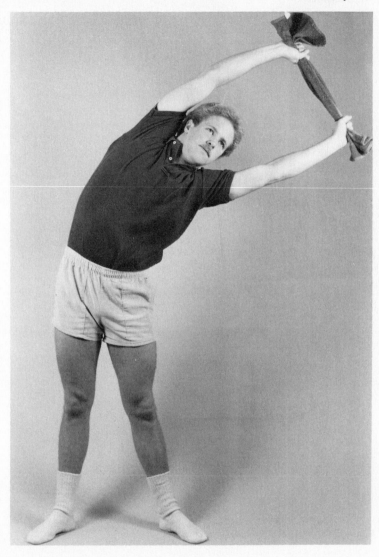

Figure 5-17. Lateral abdominal stretch.

1. Stand and hold a towel overhead with the hands about 12 inches apart, the elbows straight, and the feet 18 to 24 inches apart.
2. Bend to one side as far as possible. Keep the elbows straight.
3. Bend to the other side.

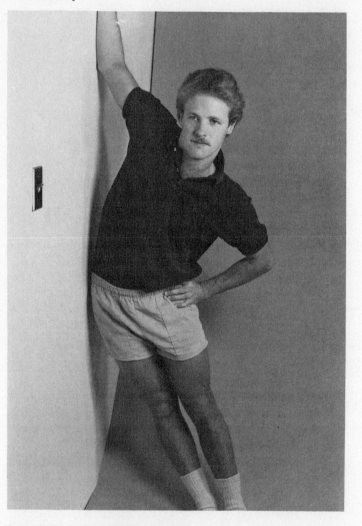

Figure 5-18. Lateral abdominal stretch.

1. Stand with the feet together and the right side toward the wall, about 18 inches from the wall.
2. Place the right hand and forearm against the wall at shoulder level. Place the heel of the left hand on the left hip.
3. Contract the abdominal and gluteal muscles and push with the hand on the hip to move the hips toward the wall. Keep the body straight and facing forward.

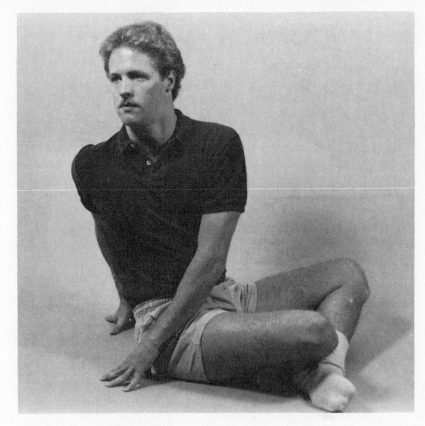

Figure 5-19. Trunk twister.

1. Sit on the floor with the legs crossed.
2. Twist the body to the right and reach to touch the floor behind the back with both hands.
3. Repeat for the left side.

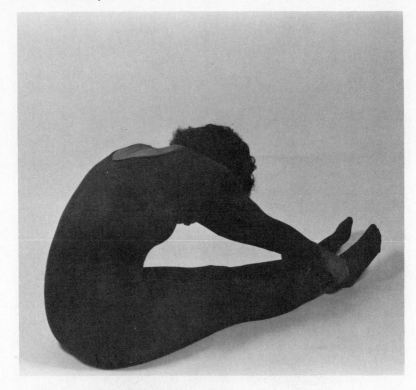

Figure 5-20. Lower back and hamstring stretch.

1. Sit on the floor with the legs straight and the feet together.
2. Bend forward and grasp the outer sides of the legs as far
   down as possible. Pull the head downward. Attempt to grasp
   the outer borders of the feet.

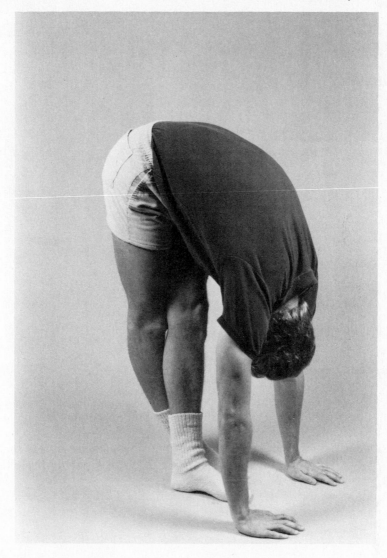

Figure 5-21. Hamstring stretch.

1. Stand with one leg crossed in front of the other and with the feet close together. The front leg holds the rear leg back and straight.
2. Slowly bend over and attempt to place the hands on the floor.
3. Repeat with each leg.

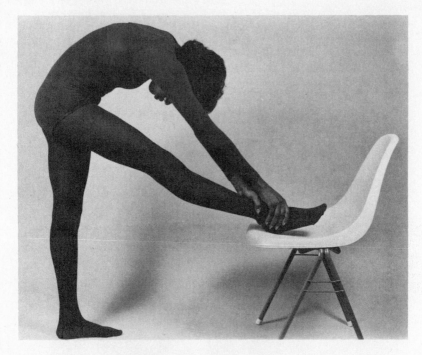

Figure 5-22.   Hamstring stretch.

1. Straighten one leg, lock the knee, and place the leg on a
   footstool.
2. Keep the other leg straight and bring the head to the knee of the
   extended leg, or toward the knee until stretch discomfort is felt.
3. Repeat with each leg.
4. Progress to the use of a chair and finally a table as
   improvement takes place.

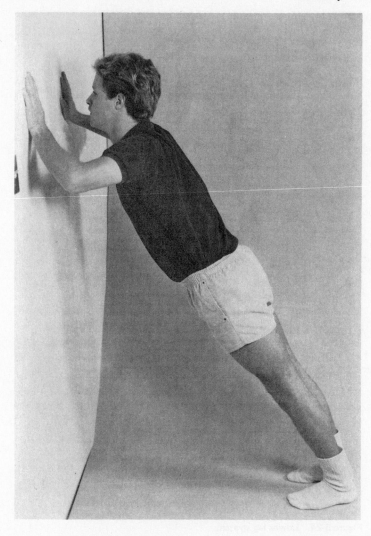

Figure 5-23. Heel cord, gastrocnemius, and soleus stretch (lower leg).

1. Stand with the face to the wall and place the palms against the wall at arm's length and at shoulder height. Keep the feet flat and the body in a straight line.
2. Lean forward and let the elbows bend until stretch discomfort is felt. Do not allow the heels to rise off the floor.

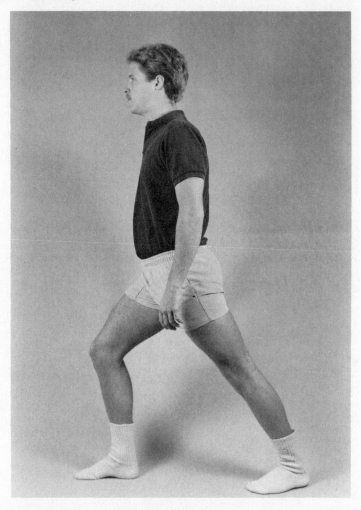

Figure 5-24. Lower leg stretch.

1. Step forward with either leg.
2. Keep the back leg straight with the foot straight ahead and the heel on the floor.
3. Bend the front leg to stretch the back leg until stretch discomfort is felt.
4. Step farther ahead with the front leg to gradually increase the distance between the feet.

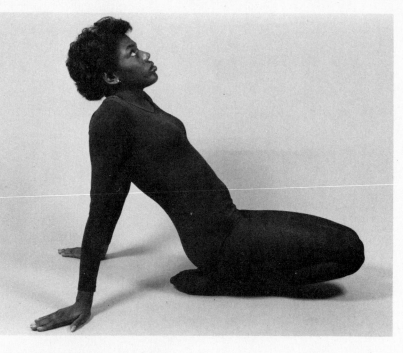

Figure 5-25. Foot and ankle stretch.

1. Sit on the feet with the toes and ankles stretched backward.
2. Balance with both hands on the floor just behind the hips.
3. Raise the knees slightly from the floor.

REFERENCES

1. deVries, H. A. *Physiology of exercise for physical education and athletics.* 2d ed. Dubuque, Iowa: William C. Brown, 1974.
2. Johnson, P. B.; Updike, W. F.; Schaefer, M.; and Stolberg, D. C. *Sport, exercise and you.* New York: Holt, Rinehart and Winston, 1975.
3. Neilson, N. P., and Jensen, C. R. *Measurement and statistics in physical education.* Belmont, Calif.: Wadsworth Publishing, 1972.
4. Rasch, P. J., and Burke, R. K. *Kinesiology and applied anatomy.* 5th ed. Philadelphia: Lea and Febiger, 1974.

KEY TERMS
Adequate diet (p. 97)
Adipose tissue (p. 96)
Basal Metabolic Rate (BMR) (p. 119)
Calorie (p. 119)
Caloric balance (p. 94)
Hyperlipidemia (p. 105)
Negative caloric balance (p. 125)
Obese (p. 94)
Overweight (p. 94)
Positive caloric balance (p. 94)

BEHAVIORAL OBJECTIVES
Upon completion of this chapter the student should be able to:
1. Define the key terms listed above.
2. List the four major reasons why individuals are overweight or obese.
3. List the four functions of adipose tissue.
4. Describe five effects of being overweight or obese.
5. Define *saturated* and *unsaturated fat, carbohydrate, protein, mineral, vitamin,* and *water* and list the functions of each of these substances.
6. State adequate percentages of carbohydrate, protein, and fat in the diet.
7. Define *cholesterol* and *triglyceride* and list the functions of these substances; state their relations to cardiovascular disease.
8. Define *fiber* and list the reasons for its inclusion in the diet.
9. Describe the problems associated with the excessive consumption of salt, sugar, and fast foods.
10. Describe ectomorph, mesomorph, and endomorph body types.
11. Describe a weight reduction plan in relation to caloric intake and exercise.

The way to a man's heart is through his stomach. How often have we all heard this statement? The prevalence of flabby waists indicates that many persons believe it. It is a tragic fact that, even though Americans enjoy the most diverse food supply in the world, a large percentage of them are overweight or obese. Public health records show that 40% to 50% of the U. S. population are **overweight:** their percentage of body fat exceeds a desirable level. One person in every five is **obese,** that is, has a body fat content that exceeds 25% (for men) or 30% (for women) of the total body weight [14, 27]. This excess weight is not limited to the older population. A 1978 Louis Harris [13] survey found that 42% of those aged 18 to 29 were overweight. Indeed, we are growing even fatter. The weight of Americans increased 5% to 7% during the past decade [2]. (See Table 6-1 for desirable weights of men and women.)

Various causes have been suggested to explain overweight and obesity, the major reasons being inactivity, overeating, emotional problems, and physiological disturbances. The last two actually involve only a small percentage of overweight people, and it is these individuals who need medical help. However, inactivity and overeating are without a doubt the major causes of excess weight in this nation's population. These two factors are related because weight gain occurs if caloric intake exceeds energy expenditure. Inactivity takes on greater significance in combination with modern dietary habits. A physically active man today eats as much as a moderately active man did a century ago, but he is less active than a sedentary man was then [27]. Indeed, the single factor most frequently held responsible for the development of excess weight and obesity is lack of exercise [19].

If caloric intake and energy expenditure are equal, there is **caloric balance,** and no weight gain occurs. However, parents often overfeed young children or allow between-meal snacks and sweets whereas they fail to encourage habits of activity. Later, during the sedentary years of adulthood, creeping obesity occurs because caloric intake exceeds metabolic use or needs, which produces a **positive caloric balance.**

Because so many Americans are overweight, there has been an array of ideas, devices, and diets that guarantee easy methods of weight control or weight reduction, and the public has annually spent millions of dollars in hope that such methods will work. There has also been much publicity concerning the value of special diets and supplements to be used with exercise programs. Unfortunately,

TABLE 6-1
METROPOLITAN LIFE INSURANCE COMPANY TABLE OF
DESIRABLE WEIGHTS (IN POUNDS) FOR MEN AND WOMEN
OF AGES 25 AND OVER (INDOOR CLOTHING)

Height (with shoes on — 1-in. heels)	Small Frame	Medium Frame	Large Frame
Men			
5 ft 2 in.	112-120	118-129	126-141
5 ft 3 in.	115-123	121-133	129-144
5 ft 4 in.	118-126	124-136	132-148
5 ft 5 in.	121-129	127-139	135-152
5 ft 6 in.	124-133	130-143	138-156
5 ft 7 in.	128-137	134-147	142-161
5 ft 8 in.	132-141	138-152	147-166
5 ft 9 in.	136-145	142-156	151-170
5 ft 10 in.	140-150	146-160	155-174
5 ft 11 in.	144-154	150-165	159-179
6 ft 0 in.	148-158	154-170	164-184
6 ft 1 in.	152-162	158-175	168-189
6 ft 2 in.	156-167	162-180	173-194
6 ft 3 in.	160-171	167-185	178-199
6 ft 4 in.	164-175	172-190	182-204
Women			
4 ft 10 in.	92- 98	96-107	104-119
4 ft 11 in.	94-101	98-110	106-122
5 ft 0 in.	96-104	101-113	109-125
5 ft 1 in.	99-107	104-116	112-128
5 ft 2 in.	102-110	107-119	115-131
5 ft 3 in.	105-113	110-122	118-134
5 ft 4 in.	108-116	113-126	121-138
5 ft 5 in.	111-119	116-130	125-142
5 ft 6 in.	114-123	120-135	129-146
5 ft 7 in.	118-127	124-139	133-150
5 ft 8 in.	122-131	128-143	137-154
5 ft 9 in.	126-135	132-147	141-158
5 ft 10 in.	130-140	136-151	145-163
5 ft 11 in.	134-144	140-155	149-168
6 ft 0 in.	138-148	144-159	153-173

Courtesy of the Metropolitan Life Insurance Company
NOTE: For those between 18 and 25, subtract 1 lb for each year under 25.

most of these methods are not based upon scientific evidence, and their promoters are more interested in money than in the health of the public.

EFFECTS OF EXCESS WEIGHT

Adipose tissue, a type of connective tissue in which many of the cells are filled with fat, is located throughout the body and serves several functions. It is found underneath the skin, where it helps reduce the loss of body heat. It also serves as a reserve food supply, which, if it is needed, can be returned to the cells by the blood and oxidized to produce energy. Adipose tissue is also present as support and protection around certain internal organs and delicate structures such as blood vessels and nerves, around joints as padding, and in the marrow of the long bones [18]. Obviously, the body needs adipose tissue and should never lack it, but serious problems can develop if there is an accumulation of excess fat. Many persons only become concerned about their weight because of their physical appearance, but there are other reasons for concern, since there is a direct relationship between fat beneath the skin and internal fat around the body organs.

Life insurance companies have stated that overweight individuals are poor risks compared with persons of normal weight, because life expectancy is shorter if there is an excessive percentage of body fat. The death rate is increased 30% for persons who are 15% to 24% overweight and as much as 80% for those who are 35% or more overweight [21].

Diseases of the heart and circulatory system are often associated with obesity. High blood pressure is twice as frequent and arteriosclerosis (hardening of the arteries) is three times more frequent in obese individuals [19]. For every 5 pounds of excess fatty tissue, 4 to 5 additional miles of blood vessels and capillaries must be formed to supply the needed blood. This places an increased burden on the heart and can contribute to the development of cardiovascular disease and diminish the chances of recovery from a heart attack.

In addition, overweight and obese individuals have more problems with their muscles and joints, more lower back problems, and a higher incidence of ruptured intervertebral discs. Excess weight creates respiratory difficulties and increases the probability that varicose veins will develop. Diabetes and problems during pregnancy occur more often, and accidental deaths are more frequent among obese individuals. Being overweight or obese is a threat to the quality and length of one's life.

FUNCTIONS OF FOOD

The term *balanced diet* designates relationships among various nutrients in an individual's diet. In the early days of nutritional science, when fewer varieties of foods were available, much emphasis was placed on balancing the carbohydrate, fat, and protein in the diet. Research has since shown that the functions of all the nutrients—vitamins, minerals, proteins, fats, carbohydrates, and water—are closely related in cellular metabolism. Hence, the term **adequate diet,** rather than *balanced diet,* should probably be used to refer to all these relationships.

The best-known and most widely recognized adequate diet consists of groups of foods that provide significant amounts or recommended daily allowances of important nutrients. Foods are grouped into the Basic Four: (1) milk and milk products, (2) meat, fish, and poultry, with nuts and legumes as alternates, (3) fruits and vegetables, and (4) breads and cereals.

There can be a positive or a negative balance of vitamins, minerals, proteins, and other nutrients as well as of Calories. It is important that the intake and the needs for all nutrients be balanced [27].

Fats

Fats, or lipids, composed of carbon and hydrogen and containing little oxygen, have the highest energy content of any food (see Table 6-2). They yield more than twice the number of Calories per gram that carbohydrates and proteins do.

The body needs moderate deposits of fat for several purposes: (1) to store a reserve fuel supply, which can provide a rich source of energy to replace carbohydrates; (2) to promote satiety or "staying power" during the slow process of digestion; (3) to enhance flavor and palatability; (4) to help provide the fat-soluble vitamins A, D, E, and K; and (5) to serve as a protective cushion for joints and some organs [4].

The classification of fats is based on the number of hydrogen atoms combined with carbon atoms. *Saturated fats* are those in which the maximum number of hydrogen atoms are attached to the carbon atoms. They harden at room temperature. Saturated animal fats are found in beef, lamb, pork, ham, butter, cream, whole milk, and cheeses made from cream and whole milk. Saturated vegetable fats are found in many solid and hydrogenated shortenings, coconut oil, cocoa butter, and palm oil (used in commercial cookies, pie fillings, and nondairy milk and cream substitutes).

Unsaturated and *polyunsaturated* fats have fewer hydrogen atoms per carbon atom than saturated fats. They are usually liquid at room temperature. They are mostly found in vegetable foods and in vegetable oils such as those derived from corn, cottonseed, safflower, sesame seed, soybean, and sunflower seed [1].

It is important to know the difference in these fats because they produce different physical effects in the body. Many nutritionists and cardiologists believe that the consumption of saturated fats increases blood cholesterol levels [6]. Studies comparing the diets and blood lipid levels of various societies support this belief. One such study observed three groups of healthy young urban Ethiopian men differing in dietary pattern [22]. The results showed striking increases in blood lipids when the diet assumed more Western characteristics. It is also believed by many nutritionists that the consumption of polyunsaturated fats tends to reduce blood cholesterol levels in many individuals [10]. It is not known how this reduction takes place. If cholesterol is taken from the blood and deposited in tissues of the body, this particular decrease in plasma cholesterol may not be beneficial. Until the reduction process is identified, it probably is best not to exceed the percentages of fats recommended by the Senate Select Committee on Nutrition and Human Needs. (See page 117.)

In addition, a diet high in saturated fats may be directly or indirectly related to the development of cancer of the colon, stomach, esophagus, breast, liver, uterus, and prostate gland. Again, studies of diets in various nations support this belief [8]. For example, the United States has a high fat intake and a high incidence of

TABLE 6-2
ENERGY SUPPLIED BY THE
THREE BASIC TYPES OF FOOD

Type of Food	Energy (Cal/gm)
Carbohydrates	4.1
Fats	9.3
Proteins	4.1

breast cancer; Japan has a low fat intake and a low incidence of breast cancer. Possibly a high intake of fats enhances the activity of cancer-producing agents, or the fats act as carriers of these agents to their site of action.

At the turn of the century, the American diet consisted of about 33% fat, but today the proportion has increased to 40% or 45%. Most nutritional experts agree that this percentage should be no more than 25% to 30% and that at least one-half to two-thirds of this total should be unsaturated and polyunsaturated fats.

Carbohydrates

Carbohydrates, which make up 45% to 50% of the American diet, are organic compounds that commonly include starches and sugars and are found in various fruits, vegetables, grains, and sweets. These compounds are broken down into a simple sugar, glucose, which the body uses as its primary source of energy. The majority of the carbohydrate intake should be in the form of starches. In the United States, however, sugar provides more than 50% of the carbohydrate intake and between 20% and 25% of the total caloric intake [20].

Proteins

Proteins are organic compounds that are needed to build and repair body tissues. They make up approximately 10% to 15% of the American diet. Red meats are excellent sources of protein, and fish, poultry, milk, grains, nuts, and legumes also provide it. The body cells do not ordinarily use protein for energy; they do so only if carbohydrate and fat supplies have been depleted. Protein is especially required during pregnancy. Even though caloric intake should decrease with age, the need for protein does not.

Minerals

The body needs *minerals* in various amounts as building materials for certain tissues and as body regulators. The more common ones are listed in Table 6-3; others include chlorine, cobalt, copper, fluorine, manganese, molybdenum, selenium, sulfur, and zinc. Minerals such as sodium and potassium can be lost through exercise, but an adequate diet will replace them without the addition of supplements.

TABLE 6-3
MINERAL SOURCES, FUNCTIONS, ADULT REQUIREMENTS, AND DEFICIENCY DISORDERS

Mineral	Sources	Functions	Adult Requirement	Deficiency Disorders
Calcium	Milk, most dairy products, shellfish, egg yolk, green vegetables	Major component of skeleton & teeth; essential for clotting of blood, normal functioning of nerve tissue	800 mg	Rickets (principal cause is deficiency of vitamin D), demineralization of bone
Iodine	Seafoods, vegetables grown on iodine-rich soils, iodized salt	Formation of thyroid hormone	0.15-0.30 mg	Goiter
Iron	Liver, lean meats, shellfish, egg yolk, dried fruits, nuts, green leafy vegetables	Oxygen transport & cellular respiration	10-15 mg	Anemia
Magnesium	Almonds, lima beans, peanuts, peas, pecans, brown rice, whole wheat, walnuts	Activation of many of body's enzymes; cardiac & skeletal muscles & nervous tissue depend on a proper balance between calcium & magnesium	300 mg	True dietary deficiency has not been reported; it can result from severe renal disease, hepatic cirrhosis, sustained losses of gastrointestinal secretions

Mineral	Sources	Functions	Amount	Comments
Phosphorus	Milk, fish, poultry, eggs	Important role in muscle energy metabolism; carbohydrate, protein, & fat metabolism; nervous-tissue metabolism; normal blood chemistry; skeletal growth; tooth development; transport of fatty acids	800 mg	Deficiency rarely found; abnormal ratio of calcium & phosphorus interferes with absorption of both elements
Potassium	Bananas, beets, molasses, sweet potatoes, green vegetables	Influence on contractility of smooth, skeletal, & cardiac muscle; affects excitability of nerve tissue	....	Deficiency rarely found, but it can cause muscular weakness & nervous irritability
Sodium	Celery, beet greens, kale, sodium chloride (salt)	Important in acid/base balance & osmotic pressure of extracellular fluids	2.5 gm	Muscular cramps, weakness, headache, interference with heat-regulating power of body

Vitamins

Vitamins function in the utilization and absorption of other nutrients and serve as components of various enzyme systems. They do not supply energy to the cells. They differ greatly in chemical composition and are found in various quantities in different foods. They must be obtained through the diet.

Vitamins are divided into two groups on the basis of their solubility. The fat-soluble vitamins, A, D, E, and K, are found in foods associated with lipids. They are normally not excreted in the urine but tend to remain stored in the body in moderate quantities. (See Table 6-4.) Owing to such reserves, the body is not absolutely dependent on a day-to-day supply. The water-soluble vitamins, B and C, are excreted in small amounts in the urine and are not stored in the body in appreciable quantities [6]. (See Table 6-5.)

Because many people believe that high doses of vitamin supplements promote good health, they annually spend millions of dollars on such supplements. Perhaps the two most advertised vitamins are C and E. Claims have been made that a vitamin C intake exceeding the minimum required amount can prevent and cure colds; however, these claims have been questioned and have not been accepted by all members of the medical profession. It has also been reported that vitamin E can prevent heart disease, reduce the serum cholesterol level, heighten sexual potency, prevent wrinkles, and perform other wonders. However, practically all the miracles claimed for vitamin E can be traced to experiments with tissue damage in vitamin-deficient animals [27]. Judgment should be used in taking large doses of these vitamins, and others as well, because they have side effects that can seriously damage the body.

Water

The most important substance in the body is *water*. It is necessary for a variety of metabolic processes, and food, oxygen, and waste products enter and leave the cells with the aid of water. In addition to other functions, it serves to lubricate the joints, cushion the spinal cord and brain, and help regulate body temperature.

A person can live for some time without food but only for a few days without water. Usually the response to thirst will maintain the body's water at a safe level, but during hot weather or after vigorous exercise, adequate water replacement may not take place. Even

TABLE 6-4
FAT-SOLUBLE VITAMIN SOURCES, FUNCTIONS, ADULT REQUIREMENTS, AND DEFICIENCY DISORDERS

Vitamin	Sources	Functions	Requirement	Deficiency Disorders
A	Liver, eggs, fishliver oils; as carotene (converted to vitamin A) in dark green & deep yellow vegetables & yellow fruits	Normal growth of epithelial tissues, normal vision, growth of bones & teeth	5,000 IU	Night blindness; rough, unhealthy skin
D	Salmon, sardines, fish, butter & cream products, liver oils, egg yolk, sunlight; artificial enrichment of suitable foods	Increase in utilization & retention of calcium & phosphorus, which ensures conditions favorable to normal mineralization of growing bone	400 IU	Inadequate intestinal absorption of calcium & phosphorus, demineralization of bone
E	Cereal seed oils, soybean oil, wheat germ oil, green leafy vegetables, legumes, nuts	Prevention of unwanted oxidation of polyunsaturated fatty acids & fat-soluble compounds	30 IU	Deficiencies rarely reported
K	Green leafy vegetables; most important source is intestinal bacterial flora, which provide adequate amount under normal circumstances	Synthesis of prothrombin by liver (blood-clotting mechanism)	Unknown	Deficiency rarely found

TABLE 6-5

WATER-SOLUBLE VITAMIN SOURCES, FUNCTIONS, ADULT REQUIREMENTS, AND DEFICIENCY DISORDERS

Vitamin	Sources	Functions	Adult Requirement	Deficiency Disorders
B_1 (thiamine)	Lean meats, eggs, whole-grain products, green leafy vegetables, nuts, legumes	Carbohydrate metabolism, nerve function	0.4 mg per 1000 Cal.	Beriberi, neuritis
B_2 (riboflavin)	Milk, cheese, meats, eggs, green leafy vegetables, whole grains, legumes	Catalysis in cellular oxidations	0.6 mg per 1000 Cal.	Fissures at angles of mouth, inflammation of tongue, visual fatigue
Niacin	Liver, meats, fish, whole grains, bread, cereals, dried peas & beans, nuts, peanut butter	Promotion of growth; important in utilization of all major nutrients	6.6 mg per 1000 Cal.	Pellagra (skin disease), nervous disorders
B_6	Liver, cereals, fish, vegetables	Protein metabolism, cell function	2 mg	Nerve inflammation, skin irritations
B_{12}	Food of animal origin, fish, milk	Formation of blood; fat & sugar metabolism; promotion of growth	3 μg	Pernicious anemia, neuritis
C (ascorbic acid)	Citrus fruits and their juices, potatoes, peppers, cabbage, tomatoes, broccoli	Metabolism of amino acids, healing of wounds, structural integrity of capillary walls, formation of intercellular substance of collagenous & fibrous tissue	50-100 mg	Scurvy, delayed healing of wounds, spongy gums, hemorrhages

following the practice of drinking five to eight glasses of fluids per day may not provide enough water. It is a good rule to drink enough water to prevent a decrease in body weight of more than 1 or 2 pounds when freely perspiring.

Diets that limit water intake should be avoided. For the purposes of weight management, however, water is Calorie-free whereas most other fluids are not.

HYPERLIPIDEMIA

Lipids (fatty materials) that are found in body tissue are also found in blood plasma. If too much of two of these lipids, cholesterol and triglyceride, is present in the blood, the condition is known as **hyperlipidemia.** It usually has no outward signs and shows only in a blood test. Numerous studies have indicated that a relation exists between hyperlipidemia and coronary heart disease. (See Chapter 2.)

The body needs cholesterol for several functions. It is a forerunner of bile salts, steroid hormones, and vitamin D. It also facilitates the absorption of fatty acids from the intestines. However, the body does not depend on dietary sources of cholesterol, because cholesterol is constantly synthesized, mainly in the liver.

As previously stated, there is a relationship between the quantity of dietary fat, its composition, and the serum cholesterol level. Table 6-6 lists the cholesterol level of certain foods. In the United States, there is wide variation in plasma cholesterol levels, but a fasting level between 150 and 200 milligrams per 100 milliliters of blood is considered healthy.

The triglyceride level can be raised by starches, sugars, saturated fats, and excessive alcohol intake, and it is often high in overweight individuals. The triglyceride level should be below 150 milligrams per 100 milliliters of blood. Many active people have less than 100 milligrams per 100 milliliters of blood.

It is not clearly understood why one individual may have hyperlipidemia while another may not, even though both have the same diet.

TABLE 6-6
CALORIC AND CHOLESTEROL VALUES OF CERTAIN FOODS

Food	Serving	Calories	Cholesterol
Vegetables			
Asparagus	10 stalks	25	N
Beans, baked	1 C	200	N
Beans, lima	1 C	150	N
Beans, green	1 C	25	N
Beets	1 C	75	N
Broccoli	1 C	45	N
Cabbage, cooked	1 C	45	N
Carrots, cooked	1 C	50	N
Celery	1 stalk	15	N
Corn	1 ear	100	N
Lettuce	1 head	50	N
Mushrooms	1 C	30	N
Peas, cooked	1 C	110	N
Potatoes, baked	1 med	125	N
Potato chips	10 med	100	N
Potatoes, french fried	6	100	M
Potatoes, sweet, baked	1 ave	200	N
Spinach, boiled	1 C	100	N
Squash	1 C	35	N
Tomato	1 med	25	N
Turnips	1 C	45	N
Animal Meats			
Bacon	2 strips	75	L
Beef, ground	4 oz	410	H
Beef, pot roast	4 oz	250	H
Beef, roast	4 oz	200	H
Beef, steak	4 oz	200	H
Ham	1 sl	100	H

NOTE: The following abbreviations are used:

ave = average	med = medium	sl = slice	sq = square
C = cup	oz = ounce	sm = small	T = tablespoon
lg = large			

The following symbols are used to represent cholesterol levels:
H = high   L = low
M = medium   N = none

TABLE 6-6, Continued

Food	Serving	Calories	Cholesterol
Ham, smoked	4 oz	450	H
Liver, beef	4 oz	150	H
Liver, calf	4 oz	160	H
Sausage	1 link	75	H
Veal chop	4 oz	150	L
Veal cutlet	4 oz	125	L
Veal roast	4 oz	250	L
Veal steak	4 oz	250	L
Chicken			
Broiled	½ med	200	L
Fried	½ med	325	M
Livers	4 oz	150	H
Pot pie	4 oz	350	M
Salad	4 oz	225	L
Turkey			
Baked	4 oz	250	L
Hash	4 oz	175	L
Soups			
Beef broth	1 C	35	L
Bean	1 C	225	L
Chicken	1 C	100	L
Chili	1 C	350	M
Tomato	1 C	100	N
Vegetable	1 C	100	N
Beverages			
Beer	8 oz	175	N
Cider	8 oz	100	N
Coffee, black	8 oz	0	N
Grapefruit juice	6 oz	75	N
Ice cream soda	1 reg	350	M
Milk, chocolate	8 oz	225	H
Orange juice	6 oz	75	N
Pineapple juice	6 oz	95	N

TABLE 6-6, Continued

Food	Serving	Calories	Cholesterol
Soft drinks	10 oz	120	N
Tea, black	1 C	0	N
Tomato juice	6 oz	50	N
Dairy Products & Eggs			
American cheese	1 oz	105	H
Butter	1 T	100	H
Cheddar cheese	1 oz	105	H
Cottage cheese	½ C	105	L
Cream	1 T	50	H
Egg, boiled	1 med	70	H
Egg, fried	1 med	100	H
Egg, scrambled	1 med	135	H
Milk, dried skim	1 T	25	L
Milk, evaporated	1 C	200	H
Milk, skim	1 C	85	L
Milk, whole	1 C	170	H
Yogurt, skim	1 C	115	L
Seafood			
Clams, steamed	12	100	L
Clams, fried	2	200	L
Flounder, fried	4 oz	150	L
Flounder, raw	4 oz	78	L
Lobster	½ C	65	M
Lobster Newburg	ave	350	H
Oysters, fried	6 med	240	M
Salmon, broiled	4 oz	140	L
Salmon, canned	½ C	200	L
Scallops	4 oz	90	L
Shrimp	10 med	100	M
Shrimp creole	ave	175	M
Shrimp, fried	10 med	315	H
Tuna, canned	3 oz	170	L
Breads and Cereals			
Biscuits, baking powder	1 lg	103	L
Biscuits, buttermilk	1 lg	90	L

TABLE 6-6, Continued

Food	Serving	Calories	Cholesterol
Bread, cinnamon	1 sl	200	L
Bread, french	1 sl	50	L
Bread, protein	1 sl	40	L
Bread, raisin	1 sl	75	N
Bread, white	1 sl	65	N
Bread, whole wheat	1 sl	65	N
English muffin	1 ave	150	L
Muffin	1 sm	125	M
Pancake	1 sm	100	M
Rice, brown	1 C	130	N
Rice, converted	1 C	130	N
Rice, white	1 C	200	N
Rolls, cinnamon	1 ave	100	M
Rolls, hot dog	1	125	N
Rolls, plain	1	100	N
Waffle	1	225	M

Fresh Fruits*

Food	Serving	Calories	Cholesterol
Apple	1 sm	75	N
Banana	1 med	100	N
Blueberries	1 C	80	N
Cantaloupe	½ med	40	N
Cherries, unpitted	1 C	95	N
Grapefruit	½ sm	50	N
Grapes	1 C	90	N
Orange	1 med	75	N
Peach	1 ave	45	N
Pear	1 ave	95	N
Pineapple	1 C	75	N
Strawberries	1 C	55	N
Watermelon	1 med slice	100	N

Candies and Nuts

Food	Serving	Calories	Cholesterol
Almonds	12	100	N
Caramel	1 med	75	M
Chocolate bar	1 sm	300	H
Fudge	1 sq	110	L

*Frozen fruits have additional calories.

TABLE 6-6, Continued

Food	Serving	Calories	Cholesterol
Peanuts	10	100	N
Peanut butter	1 T	100	N
Pecans	8	50	N
Popcorn, butter	1 C	150	M
Walnuts	4	100	N
Desserts			
Cookies, brownies	1 sq	50	H
Cookies, butter	6 sm	100	H
Cookies, chocolate chip	3 sm	65	M
Cookies, oatmeal	2 sm	50	M
Cookies, vanilla wafers	3 sm	50	L
Cake, angel food	ave	100	N
Cake, cheese	1 sm slice	350	H
Cake, chocolate	ave	250	H
Cake, pound	ave	200	H
Danish pastry	ave	200	H
Doughnut	ave	150	H
Eclair	ave	275	H
Fruitcake	1 sm	250	L
Gelatin, sweet	ave	100	N
Ice cream	1 scoop	150	M
Ice milk	1 scoop	100	L
Pie, 1 crust	ave	250	M
Pie, 2 crusts	ave	350	M
Sherbet	1 scoop	100	L
Sundae, fancy	ave	400	H
Potpourri			
Catsup	1 T	25	N
Cranberry sauce	3 T	100	N
Honey	1 T	65	N
Jam or jelly	1 T	50	N
Maple syrup	1 T	60	N
Mayonnaise	1 T	100	M
Molasses	1 T	50	N
Mustard	1 T	10	N
Pickles, dill	ave	15	N
Salad dressing, french	1 T	100	L

OTHER NUTRITIONAL CONCERNS

In addition to fats, carbohydrates, protein, minerals, vitamins, and water, there are other concerns when planning an adequate diet.

Fiber

The nondigestible component of wheat and of the roughage found in carrots, celery, apples, and other vegetables and fruits is *fiber*. It is not found in animal cells. It is unaffected by the secretions of the small intestine and passes through it undigested, and therefore does not supply nutrition; however, it provides the bulk needed to move other foods through the digestive tract.

The average American is believed to consume about 1 to 3 grams of fiber daily or approximately one-third of the amount eaten prior to the mass production of processed food [5]. According to some nutritional experts [5], the daily fiber intake should be at least 6 to 10 grams. This recommendation is based upon the following reasons:

1. Passing through the intestine like a sponge, fiber absorbs water, cholesterol, bile salts, and other materials. This hastens the propulsion of fecal material out of the bowel; and in binding with cholesterol and bile salts, the fiber possibly helps to reduce the levels of fats in the blood.

2. When fiber levels are too low, too much water is absorbed from the large intestine, causing constipation. Outpouches called diverticula may also develop in the large intestine. These outpouches are the result of the increased pressure the colon must exert to propel the slow-moving waste matter forward. When partly digested food becomes trapped in these pouches, infection may result. This inflammatory condition, called diverticulitis, requires serious surgery for about one-half million Americans each year.

3. A high-fiber diet requires more time and energy to chew. Because content is bulkier, the point of satisfaction is reached sooner, decreasing the caloric intake.

4. Low-fiber carbohydrates are more readily converted to glucose than high-fiber carbohydrates. The glucose enters the circulatory system quickly and increases the demand of the pancreas to produce insulin. This process may predispose a person to develop diabetes.

5. The evidence is not conclusive as to why, but in societies where food is less refined and more fiber is consumed, cancer of the

colon is rare. The populations of South Africa, Japan, and Finland consume much more fiber than the typical American population, and they have a significantly lower incidence of colon and rectum cancer. Mormons living in Utah also eat a high-fiber diet and experience an extremely low incidence of colon and rectum cancer [26]. The Mormons include seasonal fresh fruits, vegetables, home preserved foods, and an ample intake of grain products in their diet.

Salt

Sodium is essential for cellular function; however, only a small amount is needed by the body. Primitive herbivorous people probably consumed no more than 0.6 grams a day because plants contain very little sodium. Sodium chloride (*salt*) provides more than enough sodium intake for most Americans. It is difficult to measure exactly how much salt the average American consumes daily, but most estimates place it somewhere between 6 and 24 grams per day. Ten to 15 grams is about average [15]. This is equivalent to about four to six grams of sodium. Much of the salt is consumed in processed food, invisible. In addition, more salt is added to the food when it is cooked or prepared.

There is a major problem associated with the consumption of salt. A worldwide correlation exists between the quantity of salt ingested and the prevalence of hypertension in various populations. The Northern Japanese eat about two and one-half times as much salt as Americans, and the occurrence of hypertension is two to four times greater than it is in this nation [15]. Populations which consume a low amount of salt have a relatively low incidence of hypertension. Obese people who adopt special low-salt diets reduce their blood pressure before they reduce their body weight. Apparently, salt causes the body to retain fluid, producing an increase in the volume of blood. The increased amount of blood elevates the pressure within the blood vessels.

Salt intake can be decreased through removal of the salt shaker from the eating site, preparation of foods with other seasonings and spices, and limited intake of foods with a high salt content (e.g., canned foods, condiments, cured meats, and salted snacks).

Sugar

Most Americans consume about 125 pounds of *sugar* each year. Three-fourths of this amount is "invisible," being found in foods and beverages prepared outside the home [20]. The body needs the sugar that is obtained from the carbohydrates found in vegetables, fruits, and bread. Refined sugar does provide energy (Calories); however, it provides no protein, fat, vitamins, or fiber.

Significant problems are associated with a high sugar intake. Dental decay, excess weight, and diabetes mellitus (sugar diabetes) can occur in individuals because of excessive consumption of refined sugar. Even though it is not necessary for most people to eliminate all sugar intake, it probably would be wise to limit the amount of sugar ingestion.

Alcohol

Taken in moderation, *alcohol* does little harm. Taken in excess, however, it can be detrimental to health. In addition to the well-known serious health problems (e.g., liver and kidney impairment), there are less-known problems associated with alcohol abuse.

The Calories contained in alcohol supply no vitamins and minerals. If nutritious foods are not eaten because of excessive alcohol consumption, the individual will suffer a deficiency of vitamins and minerals. In addition, the Calories of alcohol are used for energy before food Calories. Food Calories that are not used for energy are then stored as fat, resulting in overweight. Excessive alcohol also increases the serum triglyceride level and interferes with the body's ability to utilize oxygen.

Fast Foods

According to a recent Gallop poll, 33% of this nation's adults eat out every day, and 28% of those adults eat at fast-food establishments [11]. This percentage is expected to increase during the coming years.

Fast foods really do not differ significantly from the food eaten in the average American home. That is to say, we are making the same mistake with these foods that we are making in the home. They contain too many Calories, too much fat, sugar, and too little fiber and vitamins. Most fast foods are high in protein, but few Americans are deficient in protein.

It would be a mistake to daily include them in the diet, but if eaten infrequently and as part of an adequate diet, they do not have to be avoided entirely. When it is necessary to eat fast foods often, avoiding the fried potatoes and "shakes" will decrease the fat, sugar and salt intake. Table 6-7 lists the caloric and nutritional value of many popular fast foods.

TABLE 6-7
CALORIC AND NUTRITIONAL VALUE OF FAST FOODS

	Calories	Fat Calories & Percentage of Total Calories[a]		Carbohydrate Calories & Percentage of Total Calories		Protein Calories & Percentage of Total Calories		Sodium (mg)
Hamburgers								
Burger Chef								
Big Chef	542	316	(58%)	144	(26%)	94	(17%)	—[b]
Cheeseburger	305	158	(52%)	98	(32%)	57	(19%)	—
Hamburger	258	118	(46%)	96	(37%)	44	(17%)	—
Burger King								
Cheeseburger	305	121	(40%)	116	(38%)	68	(22%)	—
Hamburger	252	81	(32%)	115	(47%)	56	(22%)	—
Whopper	660	381	(58%)	201	(30%)	78	(12%)	1083
Hot Dog	291	154	(53%)	93	(32%)	44	(15%)	—
Dairy Queen								
Big Brazier Delux	470	216	(46%)	143	(30%)	111	(24%)	—
Big Brazier Regular	457	205	(45%)	146	(32%)	106	(23%)	—
Big Brazier w/Cheese	553	271	(49%)	153	(28%)	129	(23%)	—
Brazier Dog	273	136	(50%)	93	(34%)	44	(16%)	—
Jack-In-The-Box Jumbo Jack	538	260	(48%)	180	(33%)	98	(18%)	1007
McDonald's								
Big Mac	541	280	(52%)	156	(29%)	105	(19%)	963
Cheeseburger	306	118	(39%)	123	(40%)	65	(21%)	—
Hamburger	257	83	(32%)	121	(47%)	53	(21%)	—
Quarter Pounder	418	188	(45%)	129	(31%)	101	(24%)	—
Wendy's Old Fashioned	413	205	(50%)	119	(29%)	89	(22%)	708

Sandwiches

Arby's Roast Beef	370	140 (38%)	148 (40%)	82 (22%)	869
Burger King Chopped Beef Steak	445	121 (27%)	205 (46%)	119 (27%)	966
Hardee's Roast Beef	351	158 (45%)	131 (37%)	62 (18%)	765
Roy Rogers Roast Beef	356	112 (31%)	139 (39%)	105 (29%)	610

Fish

Arthur Treacher's Original	439	251 (57%)	111 (25%)	77 (18%)	421
Burger King's Whaler	584	316 (54%)	205 (35%)	63 (11%)	968
Long John Silver's	483	251 (52%)	111 (23%)	121 (25%)	1333
McDonald's Filet-O-Fish	383	167 (44%)	156 (41%)	60 (16%)	613

Chicken

Arthur Treacher's Original	409	214 (52%)	103 (25%)	92 (22%)	580
Kentucky Fried Chicken Snack Box	405	195 (48%)	66 (17%)	44 (11%)	728

Pizza[c]

Pizza Hut					
Thin 'N Crisp/Cheese	450	136 (30%)	216 (48%)	100 (22%)	—
Thick 'N Chewy/Cheese	560	130 (23%)	285 (51%)	145 (26%)	—
Thin 'N Crisp Supreme	506	114 (23%)	262 (52%)	130 (26%)	1281

Adapted from Fast-Food Chains. Consumer Report 44:509, 512, September 1979 and H. B. Falls, A. M. Baylor, and R. K. Dishman. *Essentials of Fitness* (Philadelphia: Saunders College, 1980), pp. 297-300.

a   Percentage will not always total 100 owing to rounding off procedure.

b   Dashes indicate information not available.

c   Based on serving size of half of a 10-inch pizza.

TABLE 6-7, Continued

	Calories	Fat Calories & Percentage of Total Calories	Carbohydrate Calories & Percentage of Total Calories	Protein Calories & Percentage of Total Calories	Sodium (mg)
Taco					
Jack-In-The-Box	215	121 (56%)	70 (32%)	24 (12%)	640
Taco Bell	186	72 (39%)	56 (30%)	60 (32%)	—
French Fries[d]					
Arby's	351	—	—	—	213
Arthur Treacher's	269	—	—	—	31
Burger Chef	275	115 (42%)	143 (52%)	17 (6%)	—
Burger King	314	132 (42%)	163 (52%)	19 (6%)	78
Hardee's	287	—	—	—	306
Jack-In-The-Box	349	—	—	—	207
Long John Silver's	320	157 (49%)	150 (47%)	13 (4%)	128
McDonald's	304	140 (46%)	146 (48%)	18 (6%)	88
Roy Rogers	320	—	—	—	141
Wendy's	270	—	—	—	105

d Based on 3.5 -ounce servings. According to *Consumer Report*, the high fat content of the French fries may be due to frying the potatoes in fat or oil that is not hot enough.

Recommendations of Senate Select Committee

In 1977, after studying the health problems of America, the Senate Select Committee on Nutrition and Human Needs put forth the following dietary goals and recommendations [10].

Goals	Recommendations
1. Reduce overall fat consumption to 30% of caloric intake.	1. Decrease consumption of meat and increase consumption of poultry and fish. Substitute nonfat milk for whole milk.
2. Reduce saturated fat consumption to account for about 10% of caloric intake; and balance that with polyunsaturated and monounsaturated fats, which should account for about 10% of caloric intake each.	2. Decrease consumption of foods high in fat, and partially substitute polyunsaturated fat for saturated fat.
3. Reduce cholesterol consumption to about 300 mg a day.	3. Decrease consumption of butterfat, eggs, and other high cholesterol sources.
4. Increase carbohydrate consumption to account for 55% to 60% of caloric intake.	4. Increase consumption of fruits, vegetables, and whole grains.
5. Reduce sugar consumption to about 15% of caloric intake.	5. Decrease consumption of sugar and foods high in sugar content.
6. Reduce salt consumption to approximately 5 gm a day.	6. Decrease consumption of salt and foods high in salt content.

With six of the ten leading causes of death linked to our diet, it would seem wise to follow these recommendations.

APPRAISAL OF BODY FAT

There is no simple, objective, and truly accurate method for determining whether one is overweight or obese. Body type, total weight, and percentage of body fat are three criteria used to estimate abnormal body weight.

The morphological classification of body types includes the ectomorph, the mesomorph, and the endomorph [23]. An *ectomorph* is a slender person with a small frame: the arms and legs are small, the neck appears long, and there is little definition of muscle tissue. A *mesomorph* is an athletic-looking individual: the shoulders are broad, the hips are narrow, and there is a predominance of muscle tissue. An *endomorph* is a thick individual: the arms and legs have a rounded appearance, the chest and waist are about the same size, and the neck is thick.

Three numbers are used to designate the components of each of the three types, with 7 as the highest and 1 as the lowest rating for each. The first number refers to endomorphic, the second to meso-morphic, and the third to ectomorphic characteristics. The rating 7-1-1 designates a pure endomorph, a 1-7-1 a pure mesomorph, and 1-1-7 a pure ectomorph. It is rare to find such extreme ratings; usually there are at least two components of each type present in an individual. A 2-5-4 designation indicates fewer than average endomorphic, more than average mesomorphic, and an average number of ecto-morphic characteristics.

Body typing can be used to determine ranges of desirable body weight. (See Table 6-1.) A 5-foot-11-inch endomorph, for example, should not be expected to weigh the same as a 5-foot-11-inch ecto-morph. The technique of body typing should be performed by a qualified individual. However, a practical method for estimating one's body frame is to measure the ankle girth at the smallest point above the ankle, with the tape as tight as possible. Compare the measurement with the following standards [16]:

	Small Frame	**Medium Frame**	**Large Frame**
Men	Less than 8 inches	8 to 9.25 inches	More than 9.25 inches
Women	Less than 7.5 inches	7.5 to 8.75 inches	More than 8.75 inches

A modification of the overweight (OW) index [9] by Johnson et al. [17] can also serve as a practical method to determine whether an individual is overweight.

$$\text{OW index} = \frac{45 \times \text{body weight (lb)}}{2.5 \times \text{height (in.)} - 100}$$

Values of 100 or less indicate a satisfactory weight, and values greater than 110 indicate overweight. (See Laboratory 10.)

Desirable total body weight ranges for certain body types, how-ever, can be mistakenly interpreted if the percentages of fat and muscle tissue are not known. A range of 10% to 15% body fat for men and 15% to 20% for women is generally acceptable. Individuals with numerous mesomorphic characteristics are sometimes incorrectly considered overweight even though there is a low fat percentage due to the large amount of lean tissue.

Body-fat percentage can be estimated by underwater weighing or by measuring subcutaneous body fat with skinfold calipers. Underwater weighing is the more accurate of the two, but it requires the use of expensive laboratory equipment. Measurement with a skinfold caliper involves pinching a fold of skin between the thumb and forefinger, pulling the fold away from the underlying muscle, and applying the caliper to the fold. The thickness of the fold reflects the percentage of body fat, and therefore muscle tissue should not be included. All measurements should be taken from the right side of the body soon after awakening. Skinfold measurements are usually taken in several of the following areas: over the triceps and biceps muscles, below the shoulder blade, above the crest of the hip, in the chest and abdominal areas, and on the anterior thigh. (Figures 6-1 and 6-2 show sites for the measurement of skinfolds in females, and Figures 6-3 and 6-4 show sites in males.) The percentage of body fat can then be estimated through the use of the appropriate formula [3, 24, 25]. (See Laboratory 11.)

CALORIE NEEDS

A **Calorie**, or kilocalorie, is the measurement of a unit of energy and is defined as the amount of heat required to raise the temperature of 1 kilogram (2.2 pounds) of water to 1° C. The energy value of food is expressed in Calories. Calories are involved in all chemical reactions in the body. These reactions, referred to as *metabolism*, include processes in which food is broken down so that energy is released and those in which new substances are produced to store energy within the body.

A considerable amount of energy must be used to maintain certain vital functions—respiration, heart contraction, glandular secretions. This release of energy is called **basal metabolic rate (BMR)** and is measured when the individual is awake, reclined, and relaxed. The number of Calories required for basal metabolism varies with the age, weight, stature, hormone production, and sex of the individual, with females needing fewer than males.

Normal basal metabolism burns about 1 Calorie per hour for each kilogram of body weight. The number of Calories that a man requires per day can be estimated by multiplying his weight in pounds by 11; for women, whose BMR is about 10% lower than men's, multiply by 10 [7]. The average adult male needs approximately 1400 to 1800 Cal/day for his basal metabolism, whereas the average adult female needs approximately 1200 to 1400. Table 6-8 presents the suggested basal metabolic rates for adults.

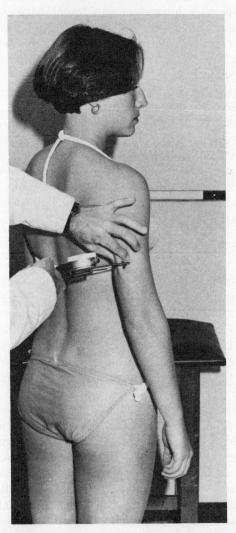

Figure 6-1. Skinfold measurement: posterior surface of arm, mid-triceps.

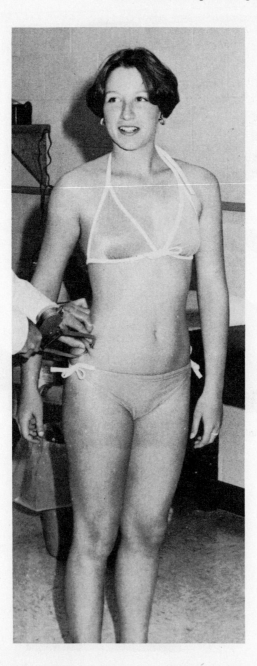

Figure 6-2. Skinfold measurement: oblique fold just above iliac crest.

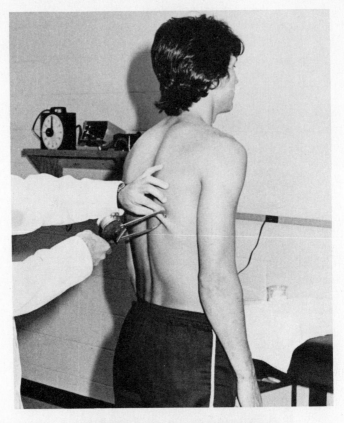

Figure 6-3. Skinfold measurement: inferior angle of scapula.

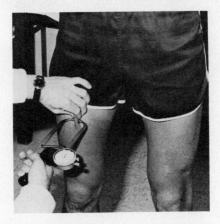

Figure 6-4. Skinfold measurement: anterior surface of mid-thigh.

TABLE 6-8
SUGGESTED BASAL METABOLIC RATES
FOR ADULTS

Height		Weight		BMR
(in.)	(cm)	(lb)	(kg)	(Cal/day)
Men				
64	163	133±11	60±5	1630
66	168	142±12	64±5	1690
68	173	151±14	69±6	1775
70	178	159±14	72±6	1815
72	183	167±15	76±7	1870
74	188	175±15	80±7	1933
76	193	182±16	83±7	1983
Women				
60	152	109±9	50±4	1399
62	158	115±9	52±4	1429
64	163	122±10	56±5	1487
66	168	129±10	59±5	1530
68	173	136±10	62±5	1572
70	178	144±11	66±5	1626
72	183	152±12	69±5	1666

Adapted with permission of the National Academy of Sciences

In proportion to body weight, BMR is highest during childhood and gradually diminishes throughout life. The decline begins during late adolescence, and its slope becomes evident at about the age of 25 in men and at about 22 in women. With increasing age, there is a gradual reduction in the number and size of functional cells; and muscle cells become fewer and are replaced by fat cells. The rate of decline in BMR is usually between 5% and 7% for each decade of life [7].

The amount of energy needed to perform functions other than basal metabolism varies in relation to daily activities. An extremely inactive individual may need only a few hundred additional Calories, whereas a large, active man may need as many as 2000 or more. Table 6-9 shows the number of Calories needed in addition to BMR.

Individuals generally become less active during the aging process. This reduction of activity together with the decline in BMR indicates that eating habits should be adjusted as one grows older to prevent gains in weight or increases in body-fat percentage. Consider Mr. Jones, whose case is based on experimental fact [7]:

When he leaves college, at age 22, he weighs 160 pounds. He is not a letterwinning athlete, but he is physically active. About 12% of his weight, just under 20 pounds, is fat. Look at Jones 35 years later, at age 57. He is proud that he weighs no more than he did when he graduated. However, he rarely exercises and has failed to maintain a regular exercise program since graduation. His body composition is radically different: he has fewer muscle cells and more fat in his fat cells. Instead of 12% fat, he now has 24%, or some 40 pounds.

And what if Jones had followed a more characteristic pattern? Suppose he had gained 20 pounds in those 35 years, a rate of only about 9 ounces per year. Those 20 pounds would be fat, so that Jones would now have about 60 pounds of fat out of a total weight of 180 pounds—he would be one-third fat. A very slight modification in eating habits or a regular exercise program would have prevented this accumulation.

It is difficult to determine how many Calories are required to maintain a constant weight. Perhaps the best method is to keep a record of what is eaten for a week during which no weight gain or loss occurs; then calculate the number of Calories (Table 6-6) and divide by 7 to determine the average daily caloric intake. (See Laboratory 12.) Compare the result with the following estimate: moderately active adults of constant weight consume the number of Calories approximately equal to 15 times their weight in pounds.

TABLE 6-9
ENERGY NEED IN ADDITION TO BMR

Activity	Energy Need (in Cal per kg of body weight)	
	Men	Women
Very light	1.5	1.3
Light	2.9	2.6
Moderate	4.3	4.1
Heavy	8.4	8.0

Adapted with permission of the National Academy of Sciences

Weight Reduction

There is no quick and easy method to reduce body weight. Extreme low-calorie diets can result in rapid weight loss, but an individual will usually return to former eating habits and regain what was lost. Diets that emphasize excessive consumption of certain foods and elimination of others often result in poor nutrition and can cause more damage than the excess weight.

Guidelines

There are certain guidelines that, if followed, should help the individual in a weight-reduction plan.

1. The body needs all types of nutrients, and the diet should consist of a balanced variety of sources. One of the dangers of Calorie counting for weight reduction is that it can lead to an inadequate intake of certain nutrients. Unless one is advised differently by a physician, the diet should consist of 55% to 60% carbohydrates, 10% to 15% protein, and 25% to 30% fat. At least one-half to two-thirds of the total fat should be unsaturated.
2. Avoid the temptation to use unsound gimmicks or diets. A reducing program should include a decrease in caloric intake and an exercise program. By combining these, the individual does not have to cut down the caloric intake as much; the loss of fat is greater, and there is an increase in the percentage of lean tissue. If the loss of weight is accomplished strictly by means of dieting, there is a loss of lean tissue as well as fat [28].
3. Weight will be lost only if there is a **negative caloric balance** (use exceeds intake). If there is a positive caloric balance (intake exceeds use), there will be a weight gain. The body stores excess Calories, whatever the source, in the form of fat.
4. The weight reduction should be a gradual one, with a loss of no more than 1 or 2 pounds per week.
5. There should be an attempt to base the amount of weight reduction on the percentage of excess body fat. However, it is difficult to determine body fat without professional help, and therefore the percentage may have to be estimated.
6. Heavy meals should be avoided. Determine the total number of Calories per day the diet will permit and divide by the number of meals. If a between-meal snack is desired, subtract the Calories it provides from the total number before dividing. For example, suppose that an individual who is on a diet of 2000

Cal/day eats a daily 200-Calorie snack. This leaves 1800 Calories for three meals, or 600 Calories each; the individual might divide it into portions of 500, 800, and 500 Calories without a heavy meal.

7. Attempt to spread the caloric intake over several meals. Studies indicate that weight reduction is more effective when the same number of Calories is consumed in three or more meals rather than one or two meals [12].

8. Dehydration or extreme water loss should be avoided. At the beginning of an exercise program, there may be a rapid initial weight reduction due to water loss, but the body will correct this water imbalance within a few days. If thirst is experienced, there should be an intake of water.

9. Attempts at spot reducing are not very effective. Exercising any group of muscles leads to a mobilization of fatty acids from fat deposits throughout the body. The public has spent much money on devices designed for such programs when general exercise programs would have been better.

10. If the reduced caloric intake is constant, the rate of weight loss will decrease as time increases due to a smaller difference between total caloric demand of the body and intake.

11. If two people are on the same caloric diet, the heavier or taller person will lose weight faster owing to a higher basal metabolic rate.

12. If a male and a female of the same age and weight are on the same caloric diet, the male will lose weight faster than the female owing to the male's higher basal metabolic rate.

Diet and Exercise

Two fallacies concerning diet and exercise often mislead the public. One is that exercise always increases the appetite and therefore results in no weight loss. The other is that exercise expends only a small number of Calories and hence, only an exhaustive exercise program can be beneficial.

The facts are, first, that an overweight individual who begins an exercise program usually makes better use of food intake and uses stored fat for energy. An underweight individual or one whose weight is correct usually has an increase in appetite as a result of exercise.

Second, the expenditure of Calories through exercise is cumulative, and weight loss is related to the duration of exercise rather than the intensity. If 250 Calories were used each day for exercise, 1750 would be used per week. Because approximately 3500 Calories equal 1 pound of body fat, this would result in the loss of 0.5 pound of body fat per week, if everything else remains equal, or 26 pounds per year. The following example is for a 145-pound woman who wishes to lose 20 pounds:

Calories deducted from diet	300
Calories used in exercise	200
Daily caloric deficit	500

$$20 \text{ lb} \times 3500 \text{ Cal/lb} = 70,000 \text{ Cal}$$
$$70,000 \text{ Cal} \div 500 \text{ deficit Cal/day} = 140 \text{ days} = 20 \text{ weeks}$$

This program takes 20 weeks to produce a loss of 20 pounds. It may actually require more days, owing to the decreasing difference between total caloric demand and intake as weight is lost.

This rate of loss may appear slow to some individuals, but it is a sensible program. It does not require starvation or extremely hard exercise. Abstaining from one 10-ounce soft drink and one average slice of pound cake amounts to avoiding the intake of 310 Calories (Table 6-6). Many desserts amount to more than 200 Calories. If this woman were to ride a bicycle for 60 minutes at 5 mph, she would expend 217 Calories. (See Table 6-10.) Furthermore, this bicycle riding would not have to be done in 60 consecutive minutes for this expenditure to take place; it could be done several times throughout the day if the total time amounted to 60 minutes. Walking for 45 minutes is another light exercise that would expend more than 200 Calories for this woman. It can be realized from this illustration and through the use of Tables 6-6 and 6-7 that a daily caloric deficit of 500 Calories is not an unrealistic goal.

Lifetime Commitment to Weight Management

It is possible for most individuals to manage their weight by eating and exercising sensibly; however, there must be a lifetime commitment to do so. A loss of weight and a reduction in the percentage of body fat does not cure a person of being overweight. Sadly, 80% or more of those who lose weight gain it back. They revert to their old eating habits and fail to maintain a regular physical exercise program. They miss the obvious—once they reach their

TABLE 6-10
ENERGY EXPENDITURE FOR VARIOUS PHYSICAL ACTIVITIES

Activity	Cal/lb			METs*
	1 Min	*15 Min*	*30 Min*	
Archery	0.0342	0.513	1.026	4.38
Basketball	0.0530	0.795	1.590	6.80
Bicycling (level road)				
5 mph	0.0250	0.375	0.750	3.21
10 mph	0.0500	0.750	1.500	6.41
13 mph	0.0720	1.080	2.160	9.23
Bowling	0.0486	0.729	1.458	6.23
Calisthenics	0.0333	0.795	1.590	4.27
Golf (walking)	0.0360	0.540	1.080	4.62
Handball	0.0630	0.945	1.890	8.08
Hiking	0.0420	0.630	1.260	5.38
Paddleball	0.0690	1.035	2.070	8.85
Ping-Pong	0.0304	0.456	0.912	3.90
Running (cross country)	0.0740	1.110	2.220	9.49
Running (level track)				
4.5 mph (13:30 min/mi)	0.0630	0.945	1.890	8.08
5.0 mph (12:00 min/mi)	0.0667	0.999	1.999	8.55
5.5 mph (11:00 min/mi)	0.0711	1.067	2.133	9.12
6.0 mph (10:00 min/mi)	0.0790	1.185	2.370	10.13
7.0 mph (8:30 min/mi)	0.0933	1.399	2.799	11.96
8.7 mph (6.54 min/mi)	0.1031	1.547	3.094	13.22
10.0 mph (6:00 min/mi)	0.1066	1.599	3.198	13.67
12.0 mph (5:00 min/mi)	0.1311	1.967	3.933	16.81
Running (sprints)	0.1552	2.328	4.656	19.90
Squash	0.0691	1.037	2.074	8.86
Stationary running				
70-80 counts/min	0.0780	1.170	2.340	10.00
140 counts/min	0.1622	2.433	4.866	20.79

Adapted from C. F. Consolazio, R. E. Johnson, and L. J. Pecora, *Physiological measurements of metabolic functions in man* (New York: McGraw-Hill, 1963), pp. 331-32.
NOTE: The number of calories expended in any activity can be obtained by multiplying the number of calories per minute per pound by your weight and by the number of minutes the activity is performed.
*Based on an average caloric consumption of 1.2 Cal/min for a 154-lb man sitting at rest.

TABLE 6-10, Continued

Activity	Cal/lb			METs*
	1 Min	*15 Min*	*30 Min*	
Swimming (pleasure)	0.0724	1.086	2.172	9.28
Breast stroke (20 yd/min)	0.0319	0.479	0.958	4.09
Breast stroke (40 yd/min)	0.0639	0.959	1.918	8.19
Back stroke (25 yd/min)	0.0252	0.378	0.756	3.23
Back stroke (35 yd/min)	0.0454	0.681	1.362	5.82
Side stroke (40 yd/min)	0.0554	0.831	1.662	7.10
Crawl (45 yd/min)	0.0580	0.870	1.740	7.44
Crawl (55 yd/min)	0.0706	1.059	2.118	9.05
Tennis	0.0460	0.690	1.380	5.90
Volleyball	0.0233	0.350	0.699	2.99
Walking (level ground)				
2.27 mph (26:26 min/mi)	0.0233	0.350	0.700	2.99
3.20 mph (18:45 min/mi)	0.0313	0.470	0.940	4.01
3.50 mph (17:09 min/mi)	0.0332	0.498	0.996	4.26
4.47 mph (13:25 min/mi)	0.0524	0.786	1.572	6.72
4.60 mph (13:03 min/mi)	0.0551	0.827	1.654	7.06
5.18 mph (11:35 min/mi)	0.0627	0.941	1.882	8.04
5.80 mph (10:21 min/mi)	0.0756	1.134	2.268	9.69

desired weight, they can eat more than when on their diet; however, to keep their weight down, they must eat less than before. They must experience permanent behavioral change in their eating and activity habits.

REFERENCES

1. American Heart Association. *The way to a man's heart.* New York: American Heart Association, 1972.
2. Bray, G. The nutritional message must be spread. *Journal of the American Medical Association* 241:1320–1321, 1979.
3. Brozek, J.; Grande, F.; Anderson, J. T.; and Keys, A. Densitometric analysis of body composition: Revision of some quantitative assumptions. *Annals of the New York Academy of Science* 110:113–140, 1963.
4. Bucher, C. A.; Olsen, E. A.; and Willgoose, C. E. *The foundations of health.* New York: Appleton-Century-Crofts, 1967.

5. Burkitt, D. P. The link between low-fiber diets and diseases. In *Readings in health 80/81.* Guilford, Conn.:Dushkin Publishing Group, 1980.

6. Burton, B. T. *The Heinz handbook of nutrition.* New York: McGraw-Hill, 1965.

7. Deutsch, R. M. *The family guide to better food and better health.* Des Moines: Meredith Corporation, 1971.

8. Eckholm, E., and Record, F. The affluent diet—a worldwide health hazard. In *Readings in health 80/81.* Guilford, Conn.: Dushkin Publishing Group, 1980.

9. Fabry, P.; Hejl, Z.; Fodor, J.; Braun, T.; and Zvolankova, K. The frequency of meals: Its relation to overweight, hypercholesterolemia, and decreased glucose tolerance. *Lancet* 2:614–615, 1964.

10 Falls, H. B.; Baylor, A. M.; and Dishman, R. K. *Essentials of fitness.* Philadelphia: Saunders College, 1980.

11. Fast-food chains. *Consumer Report* 44:508–513, 1979.

12. Guggenheim, F. G. Basic consideration in the treatment of obesity. *Medical Clinics of North America* 61:781–796, 1977.

13. Harris, L., and Associates. *Health maintenance survey.* Newport Beach, Calif.: Pacific Mutual Life Insurance Company, 1978.

14. Hockey, R. V. *Physical fitness.* 2d ed. St. Louis: C. V. Mosby, 1973.

15. Jacobson, M. The deadly white powder. In *Readings in health 80/81.* Guilford, Conn.: Dushkin Publishing Group, 1980.

16. Johnson, P. B. *So you really want to lose weight?* Toledo: The University of Toledo, 1972. In P. B. Johnson; W. F. Updike; M. Schaefer; and D. C. Stolberg. *Sport, exercise and you.* New York: Holt, Rinehart and Winston, 1975.

17. Johnson, P. B.; Updike, W. F.; Schaefer, M.; and Stolberg, D. C. *Sport, exercise and you.* New York: Holt, Rinehart and Winston, 1975.

18. Kimber, D. C.; Gray, C. E.; Stackpole, C. C.; and Leawell, L. C. *Anatomy and physiology.* New York: Macmillan, 1966.

19. Mayer, J. *Overweight: Causes, cost and control.* Englewood Cliffs, N.J.: Prentice-Hall, 1968.

20. Mayer, J. The bitter truth about sugar. In *Readings in health 80/81.* Guilford, Conn.: Dushkin Publishing Group, 1980.

21. Neal, K. G. *Knowledge of health series.* Long Beach, Calif.: ELOT Publishing, 1975.

22. Ostwald, R., and Gebre-Medhin, M. Westernization of diet and serum lipids in Ethiopians. *The American Journal of Clinical Nutrition* 31:1028–1040, 1978.

23. Sheldon, W.; Stevens, S. S.; and Tucker, W. B. *The varieties of human physique.* Darien, Conn.:Hafner, 1970.

24. Sloan, A. W. Estimation of body fat in young men. *Journal of Applied Physiology* 23:311–315, 1967.

25. Sloan, A. W.; Burt, J. J.; and Blyth, C. S. Estimation of body fat in young women. *Journal of Applied Physiology* 17:967–970, 1962.

26. Upton, A. C. Status of the diet, nutrition and cancer program. Statement before the Subcommittee on Nutrition, Senate Committee on Agriculture, Nutrition and Forestry, October 2, 1979.

27. White, P. L. and Selvy, N. *Let's talk about food.* Acton, Mass.: Publishing Sciences Group, 1974.

28. Zuti, W. B., and Golding, L. A. Comparing diet and exercise as weight reduction tools. *The Physician and Sportsmedicine* 4 (1):49–53, 1973.

KEY TERMS

Catecholamines (p. 135)
Depression (p. 140)
Homeostatic balance (p. 134)
Relaxation (p. 137)
Stress (p. 134)
Stressor (p. 134)
Sympathetic nervous system (p. 134)
Tension (p. 135)

BEHAVIORAL OBJECTIVES

Upon completion of this chapter the student should be able to:

1. Define the key terms listed above.
2. Describe six body changes promoted by the sympathetic nervous system and the adrenal glands in response to a stressor.
3. Define epinephrine and norepinephrine and describe the effects of these substances.
4. Describe the tense individual.
5. List eight stress-related diseases and disorders.
6. Describe the role of exercise in the prevention of stress-related diseases.
7. Determine whether he or she is a tense individual.
8. Release tension through a relaxation technique.
9. Describe the depressed individual.
10. Describe the role of exercise in the treatment of depression.

CHAPTER SEVEN
Stress and Depression

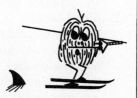

If the **homeostatic balance** (physiological equilibrium) of the body is disturbed, the individual experiences **stress**. Psychological as well as physiological conditions can promote stress, but, whatever the cause, the body does not differentiate among the **stressors**. The reaction to emotional stress appears to be physiologically identical to the reaction induced by physical stress. It continues to exist in the body until homeostatic balance is restored.

Not everyone reacts the same to stress. Some individuals thrive on stress and actually rise to the occasion to function better mentally and physically; many top executives of major businesses fall in this category. In addition, certain individuals do not react emotionally to experiences that can be considered stressful. Their personalities appear to remain calm. However, others react strongly and become emotionally and physically disturbed. These people often have physical problems or disorders. The difference in the reactions of people to an emotional crisis is often due to the various ways in which they perceive stress. Some magnify the significance of an experience, whereas others are able to perceive that the experience may not be important.

Selye, a Canadian physician and endocrinologist, describes three stages the body goes through during stress [18]. Initially, during the alarm reaction stage, the body reacts to stress. Changes in body chemistry take place to prepare the body for the stressful experience. This stage is followed by the resistance state, in which the body attempts to adapt to the stress. If no adaptation takes place, the exhaustive stage follows, in which physical disorders, or possibly even death, are experienced.

BODY CHANGES

Sudden emotions of fear, anger, or excitement stimulate the **sympathetic nervous system** and the *adrenal glands* to instant action. The sympathetic nervous system produces the following changes in the body [1].

1. The heart rate and stroke volume are increased, which results in an increased cardiac output.
2. Blood vessels in the skin, kidneys, and most internal organs become constricted, which decreases the blood flow to these areas; blood vessels in the skeletal muscles become dilated, which increases the flow to them.
3. Systolic blood pressure and the volume of blood circulating per minute are increased.

4. Secretions of the digestive glands and contractions of the small intestine are decreased and thus there is decreased digestion.
5. Liver glycogenolysis (breakdown of glycogen to glucose) is increased, which results in more blood glucose.
6. The breakdown of adipose-tissue triglyceride is increased.
7. The rate of ventilation is increased.
8. Muscle **tension** is increased.

There is also a rapid and marked rise in the amount of epinephrine (adrenaline) and norepinephrine secreted by the adrenal medulla. These two important secretions, known as **catecholamines,** help to increase and prolong the responses of the sympathetic nervous system. Epinephrine accelerates the rate and increases the strength of heart contraction, dilates coronary and skeletal muscle blood vessels, and constricts vessels in many other body organs; thus it raises blood pressure and redirects blood flow to areas with increased metabolic needs. Norepinephrine is almost exclusively a vasoconstrictor for the small blood vessels of muscle tissue (*peripheral circulation*) and plays a minor role in the increase in cardiac pumping.

Stress also initiates a series of reactions that stimulate the adrenal cortex to release the hormone cortisol. The functions of cortisol are as follows [20]:

1. Stimulation of protein catabolism
2. Stimulation of the liver to convert amino acids to glucose
3. Inhibition of the oxidation of glucose by many body cells, but not by the brain

These body changes promoted by the sympathetic nervous system and the adrenal glands are ideally suited to cope with stressful experiences. When primitive humans were faced with emotionally exciting and physically demanding situations, they usually had to be prepared to fight for their lives or to run to save themselves. Either choice required action and placed demands upon the body. The sympathetic nervous system helped the cardiovascular and respiratory systems to supply oxygen and nutrients to the body cells and to remove waste products. The effects of cortisol enabled people to forego eating for a lengthy period, which they often had to do on occasions of danger. In addition, the amino acids liberated by the catabolism of body protein provided energy and assisted in tissue repair if injury occurred. Today, these body changes continue to take place when people are confronted with stress. Recent evidence suggests that the secretion of almost every known hormone can be influenced by stress [20].

Emotional conflicts brought on by the many turmoils of our present society stimulate a person's glands, which prepare the body for a stressful experience. However, urban civilization makes it virtually impossible to relieve the tensions within the body, because people are not provided with the motivation and opportunity for, or the social approval of, the vigorous activities needed to neutralize hormone secretions. Modern society has made the fight-or-flight concept obsolete, but it has not changed the autonomic nervous system's response to stress. It is very possible that failure to understand this response contributes to the development of stress-induced diseases.

THE TENSE INDIVIDUAL

The muscles are arranged in pairs around each joint. As one member of the pair contracts, the other should relax. If the opposing muscle is under tension, it does not relax but resists movement, which results in wasted energy, further fatigue, and increased tension. The tense individual, expending vast amounts of energy without producing results other than fatigue, is therefore not a physically efficient person and is often very tired [13].

The habitually tense individual seeks to release tension in physical actions that are in no way related to the problem created by the tension—drumming the fingers on the table aimlessly or forcibly to express irritation; continually moving in the chair in attempts to find a comfortable position; twisting a lock of hair, scratching the scalp, or pulling at an ear; gripping a pencil until the fingers become numb; twisting a handkerchief or clasping the hands in a deathlike grip; twitching the face or assuming expressions of intense concentration, grinding the teeth, and shrugging the shoulders. Sitting "motionless," the tense individual twists a ring about the finger, crosses and uncrosses the legs, and wraps the feet around each other. Movement and posture appear stiff. Such a person complains of being tired, worries, and easily becomes angry or frustrated if faced with a problem for which there is no immediate solution [12]. (See Laboratory 13.)

STRESS-RELATED DISEASES AND DISORDERS

Emotional stress without meaningful physical movement has very detrimental effects on the body. It increases the levels of fatty acids in the bloodstream, and hence it is related to atherosclerotic problems [9]. Prolonged tension, if frequently repeated, can lead to insomnia, colitis, and hypertension. Digestion is inhibited and acid enters the stomach, which leads to ulcers. Constipation, high serum cholesterol, and shortened time of blood coagulation are also consequences of emotional stress without physical movement. The muscle tightness that usually accompanies unpleasant emotions can create back, neck, chest, and stomach pains. Other symptoms of stress include headache, blurred vision, loss of appetite, and depression. Indeed, Selye's theory of stress postulates that almost any disease can be caused by emotional tension.

TECHNIQUES FOR RELAXATION

Relaxation is a conscious release of muscular tension. It is a skill that is based on an awareness of the presence of tension, and it is one that is not easily performed by many individuals. These individuals must learn to relax in much the same way that they would learn any other motor skill [19].

Various relaxation techniques have been reported to be successful in the release of tension. Benson [4] proposed the following technique:

1. Sit quietly in a comfortable position and close the eyes.
2. Beginning at the feet and progressing to the head, relax all the muscles.
3. Breathe through the nose. Each time you breathe out, silently say the word *one.* Breathe easily and naturally.
4. Continue for 10 to 20 minutes. You may occasionally check the time, but do not use an alarm. When you finish, sit quietly for several minutes.
5. Maintain a positive attitude and permit relaxation to occur at its own pace. When distracting thoughts occur, try to ignore them by not dwelling upon them, and continue to repeat the word *one.*

Arnheim et al. [2] reported a more involved relaxation technique.

1. Assume a supine position on a firm mat with each body curve (i.e., the neck, elbows, lower back, and knees) comfortably supported by a pillow or a towel. The arms should be spread so that they do not contact the clothing or the body. Take five deep breaths; inhale and exhale slowly.

2. Curl the toes down and point the feet downward. Do not bite down hard with the teeth or hold the breath. Relax. Try to relax all other parts as you tense one area of the body.

3. Curl the toes and the feet back toward the head. Breathe easily and relax.

4. Press down against the floor with the heels and attempt to curl the legs backward. Relax.

5. Straighten the legs to full extension. Let go and breathe easily.

6. Draw the thighs up to a bent position and raise the heels about 3 in. off the floor. Tension should be felt in the bend of the hip. Return slowly to the starting position and relax.

7. Forcibly rotate the thighs outward. Feel the tension in the outer hip region. Relax.

8. Rotate the thighs inward. Feel the tension deep in the inner thighs. Relax slowly and let the thighs again rotate outward.

9. Squeeze the buttocks together tightly and tilt the hips backward. Tension should be felt in the buttocks and also in the lower back. Relax.

10. Tighten the abdominal muscles and flatten the lower back. Tension should be felt in both areas. Relax.

11. Inhale and exhale slowly and deeply three times. Return to normal quiet breathing.

12. Press the head back and lift the upper back off the floor. The tension should be felt in the back of the neck and upper back. Relax.

13. Squeeze the shoulder blades together. Tension should be felt in the back of the shoulders. Relax.

14. Leaving the arms in their resting position, lift and roll the shoulders inward so that tension is felt in the front of the chest. Relax.

15. Spread and clinch the fingers of both hands three times. Relax.

16. Make tight fists with both hands and slowly curl the wrists back, forward, and to both sides. Allow the fingers and thumbs to open gradually and relax.

17. Make tight fists with both hands and slowly flex the forearm against the upper arm. At the same time, lift the arm at the shoulder. Slowly uncurl the arms and return them to their original resting position. Relax.

18. Make tight fists with both hands, stiffen the arms, and press hard against the floor. Hold the pressure for 30 seconds. Slowly relax.

19. Shrug the right shoulder. Bend the head sideward and touch the ear to the elevated shoulder. Slowly relax.

20. Repeat step 19 with the left shoulder.
21. Bend the head forward and touch the chin to the chest. Slowly relax.
22. Lift the eyebrows upward and wrinkle the forehead. Let the face go blank.
23. Close the eyelids tightly and wrinkle the nose. Relax the face slowly.
24. Open the mouth widely as if to yawn. Slowly relax.
25. Bite down hard and then show the teeth in a forced smile. Slowly relax.
26. Pucker the lips in a whistle position. Slowly relax.
27. Push the tongue hard against the roof of the mouth. Relax. Perform this three times.
28. Move slowly and take any position desired. Relax and rest.

With practice, either of the above techniques can be successful in the promotion of relaxation. Individuals who have difficulty in the attainment of a relaxed state should use a technique that is successful for them. (See Laboratory 14.)

In a study of 75 adult men, Bahrke and Morgan [3] compared the reduction of tension through exercise, quiet rest, and performance of Benson's Relaxation technique. All three treatments were performed for 20 minutes and were equally effective in reducing tension. Possibly, for the treatment of stress, just "getting away from it all" may be just as important as any physiological changes which may take place through exercise.

STRESS AND PHYSICAL EXERCISE

People are designed to be physically active, and many experts believe that movement can help prevent stress-related diseases and problems. Some studies indicate that fat is cleared more rapidly from the blood after exercise and that a physical training program increases this effect; this serves to prevent atherosclerosis [21].

Michael [14] found that moderate exercise actually provides a mild type of stress for the adrenal glands, which helps to condition and fortify them so that they can manage severe stresses more effectively. The increased adrenal activity that results from repeated exercise seems to cause the formation of greater reserves of steroids, which are suitable for counteracting stress.

Other studies have indicated that repeated physical exercise decreases catecholamine uptake by the trained heart [17]. The heart responds to catecholamines with an increased pulse rate and an augmented coronary blood flow. However, the trained heart is more efficient in this response and more sensitive to the increased oxygen need, and thus it wastes less myocardial oxygen.

Studies involving mentally ill patients have verified that sports and moderate physical activity have value in the release of tension. DeVries [7] concluded that rhythmic exercise, such as walking, jogging, bicycling, and bench-stepping, with durations of 5 to 30 minutes and intensities of 30% to 60% of maximum heart rate, promoted significant relaxation for the tense individual. Also, through concentration on the game and on the opponent, tennis players, handball players, and participants in similar activities find a mental diversion that provides their worried minds with a new set of problems to solve; solutions to these problems, however, can be found in a short space of time. Habitual worry or anxiety is temporarily forgotten, and physical tensions arising from these concerns are released [6]. As previously reported, Bahrke and Morgan [3] found exercise, quiet rest, and Benson's Relaxation technique equally effective in reducing tension; however, according to the researchers, tension reduction following exercise can be sustained for a longer period than that of the other two treatments.

Selye [18] classifies exercise as a potent stressor. In the first stage, the body responds to the demands of exercise. Through training and progressive amounts of reasonable exercise, an efficient response results, and the exhaustion phase of stress is deterred. Selye suggests that an individual who exercises regularly should be better prepared to resist other stressors and that stressful situations are not as dangerous to a physically conditioned individual as to a sedentary individual.

Socially acceptable outlets for natural aggressive drives provide important physical and emotional benefits. Anger, hate, and frustration, often excluded by society from open expression, can be transformed into running, swimming, tennis, golf, or many other forms of physical activity, and this results in a healthier and happier life.

DEPRESSION

Depression is a very common disorder. Up to 15 million Americans annually experience the symptoms of depression [8]. Sometimes called the common cold of mental illness, depression underlies many of the physical complaints physicians are asked to treat, and it hospitalizes hundreds of thousands of people each year. It also is responsible for the high suicide rate among teenagers.

Depression usually relates to a loss, a disappointment, or the failure to manage stress. When depressed, the individual becomes a captive of bad moods and is not able to remain in a good or pleasant mood.

Such factors as one's job, homemaking responsibilities, financial obligations, parental responsibilities, the stress of marriage or being single, unhealthy lifestyles, decline in moral values, not knowing what is expected for adequate performance of a role or task, and the failure to fulfill personal expectations contribute to depression. The more factors experienced, the greater the chances of depression. The traits most often exhibited by depressed individuals are poor appetite, a lonely feeling, tendency to withdraw, little interest in other people or things, trouble falling asleep or staying asleep, little energy, preoccupation with unhappiness, and thoughts about suicide.

DEPRESSION AND PHYSICAL EXERCISE

Drugs, electroshock, sleep deprivation, and counseling have been used to treat extreme cases of depression; however, with increasing frequency medical authorities are prescribing physical exercise programs as therapy for mild to moderate depression [5, 9, 10, 15]. They are impressed by the benefits that many depressed individuals obtain from extended, systematic periods of regular physical activity such as walking, jogging, swimming, bicycling, tennis, and racquetball. Males and females, young and old, have experienced a significant reduction in depression through regular exercise. Robert Brown, University of Virginia [10], and Thaddeus Kostrubala, author of The Joy of Running [11], are psychiatrists who prescribe exercise as treatment for depression. Because exercise is such effective therapy, they do not prescribe antidepressant drugs as freely as they once did.

Research has failed to show how exercise relieves depression. Some medical authorities believe that biochemical changes in the brain and other nerve tissues may help move a depressed individual toward a more functional state, but other, simpler explanations have also been proposed.

1. The body and mind do not operate on different levels, independent of each other. If the body breaks down, the mind suffers; if the body is strengthened, the mind is too [12].

2. Exercise may be antagonistic to depression. Because the way we feel in our mind can make us feel bad physically, it can also work the other way [12].
3. Physical activity provides depressed individuals the satisfaction of mastering what they believe to be difficult. Through exercise they can meet and accomplish a goal. Fulfilling a goal can help individuals to like themselves better.
4. Walking, running, bicycling, or other similar activities may serve to stimulate daydreaming and unconscious mind release. The mind is allowed to "spin" and relax, causing blue moods to leave. The exercise environment may be an important part of the healing process. The smell, touch, and feel of the outdoors provide distractions that prevent the depressed individual from concentrating on any problems.

How Much Exercise?

The antidepressant effect of exercise may depend on the type, intensity, duration, and frequency of the exercise. Brown et al. [5] demonstrated that walking three miles within 45 minutes several times a week relieved depression; and in comparing the influence of tennis and jogging on depression, they found both to provide effective relief. Moreover, jogging five days a week for ten weeks caused a greater reduction in depression than playing tennis or jogging for three days. Brown et al. concluded that there is more therapeutic value in vigorous physical activities. Kostrubala's patients also experienced better antidepressant effects with running programs of at least moderate intensity, duration, and frequency [11].

It is probable that the antidepressant benefits of exercise best occur when the exercise involves rhythmic movement of large muscles and is performed three to five times a week at moderate intensity. Whether performed alone or with someone is an individual decision.

Negative Addiction

Morgan [16] proposed that it is possible to become negatively addicted to exercise. Negative addiction is present if two basic requirements are met. First, the individual believes that he or she cannot live without daily exercise; and second, if deprived of exercise, the individual experiences withdrawal symptoms (e.g., depression, anxiety, and irritability). Hard-core exercise addicts exercise despite injury and give their daily exercise higher priority than job, family, or friends.

There can be no doubt that regular exercise can provide many benefits, but an exercise program must be kept in perspective from a vocational, social, physiological, and psychological standpoint. Joggers, swimmers, bicyclists, etc., should control the exercise experience rather than let the program control them. Exercise is a means to an end—the achievement of physical and mental health.

REFERENCES

1. Anthony, C. P., and Kolthoff, N. J. *Anatomy and physiology.* 9th ed. St. Louis: C. V. Mosby, 1975.
2. Arnheim, D. D.; Auxter, D.; and Crowe, W. C. *Principles and methods of adapted physical education.* St. Louis: C. V. Mosby, 1969.
3. Bahrke, M. S., and Morgan, W. P. Anxiety reduction following exercise and meditation. *Cognitive Therapy and Research* 2:323–333, 1978.
4. Benson, H. *The relaxation response.* New York: William Morrow and Company, 1975.
5. Brown, R. S.; Ramirez, D. E.; and Taub, J. M. The prescription of exercise for depression. *The Physician and Sportsmedicine* 6 (12):34–45, 1978.
6. Byrd, O. Studies on the psychological values of lifetime sports. *Journal of Health, Physical Education, Recreation* 38:35–36, November–December 1967.
7. deVries, H. A. Physical education, adult fitness programs: Does physical activity promote relaxation? *Journal of Physical Education and Recreation* 46 (7):53–54, 1975.
8. Falls, H. B.; Baylor, A. M.; and Dishman, R. K. *Essentials of fitness.* Philadelphia: Saunders College, 1980.
9. Folkins, C. H.; Lynch, S.; and Gardner, M. M. Psychological fitness as a function of physical fitness. *Archives of Physical Medicine and Rehabilitation* 53:503–508, 1972.
10. Higdon, H. Can running put mental patients on their feet? *Runner's World* 13 (1):36–43, 1978.
11. Kostrubala, T. *The joy of running.* New York: Pocket Books, 1977.
12. Martin, J. In activity therapy, patients literally move toward mental health. *The Physician and Sportsmedicine* 5 (7):84–89, 1977.
13. Methany, E. *Body dynamics.* New York: McGraw-Hill, 1952.
14. Michael, E. D. Stress adaptation through exercise. *Research Quarterly* 28:50–54, 1957.
15. Morgan, W.P. A pilot investigation of physical working capacity in depressed and nondepressed psychiatric males. *Research Quarterly* 40:859–860, 1969.
16. ———. Negative addiction in runners. *The Physician and Sports-medicine* 7 (2):56–70, 1979.
17. President's Council on Physical Fitness and Sports. Effects of chronic exercise on cardio-vascular function. *Physical Fitness Research Digest,* edited by H. H. Clark, series 2, no. 3, July 1972.
18. Selye, H. *The stress of life.* New York: McGraw-Hill, 1956.

19. Scott, M. A. *Analysis of human motion.* 2d ed. New York:Appleton-Century-Crofts, 1963.
20. Vander, A. J.; Sherman, J. H.; and Luciano, D. S. *Human physiology—the mechanism of body function.* 2d ed. New York: McGraw-Hill, 1975.
21. Watt, J. Exercise and heart disease—related fields of research. In *Exercise and Fitness,* edited by S. C. Staley, T. K. Cureton, L. J. Huelster, and A. J. Barry. Chicago: Athletic Institute, 1960.

KEY TERMS
Accelerator nerve (p. 147)
Aorta (p. 146)
Atria (p. 146)
Atrioventricular (A-V) node (p. 148)
Atrioventricular (A-V) valve (p. 146)
Bundle of His (p. 148)
Chordae tendineae (p. 146)
Diastasis (p. 149)
Diastole (p. 149)
Interventricular septum (p. 148)
Murmurs (p. 150)
Myocardium (p. 146)
Pulmonary artery (p. 146)
Pulmonary veins (p. 146)
Purkinje fibers (p. 148)
Semilunar valves (p. 146)
Sinoatrial (S-A) node (p. 148)
Systole (p. 149)
Vagus nerve (p. 147)
Venae cavae (p. 146)
Ventricles (p. 146)

BEHAVIORAL OBJECTIVES
Upon completion of this chapter, the student should be able to:
1. Define the key terms.
2. Make a schematic diagram of the heart and label the following structures:
    a. Right and left atria
    b. Right and left ventricles
    c. Interventricular septum
    d. Myocardium
    e. Pulmonary artery, pulmonary veins
    f. Aorta
    g. Superior and inferior venae cavae
    h. Mitral and tricuspid valves
    i. Pulmonary and aortic valves
3. Trace blood flow from right atrium to aorta; list in order the structures passed.
4. Identify basic events of the cardiac cycle and causes of the first and second heart sounds.
5. List normal values for resting heart rate, systolic blood pressure, diastolic blood pressure, stroke volume, and cardiac output.
6. List maximum normal values for heart rate and systolic blood pressure.

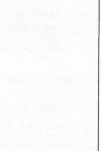

HEART

BLOOD

The ability of one's circulorespiratory system to deliver blood with its oxygen to active muscle tissue appears, at present, to be the most important limitation of exercise. Although there is a high rate of energy turnover during cardiac work, the mechanical efficiency of the heart per beat is very low. Nevertheless, the amount of work accomplished by this small organ, without cessation or breakdown, is astonishing. It has been calculated that the work performed by a normal heart during one's lifetime is the equivalent of lifting a 30-ton weight to a height of 30,000 feet [2].

BASIC STRUCTURE

As can be seen in Figure 8-1, the heart is a hollow organ composed of four chambers. The upper chambers are identified as the left and right **atria,** and the lower chambers are the **ventricles. Atrioventricular (A-V) valves** (mitral and tricuspid) connect the atria with the ventricles. Attached to the cusps of these valves are tendinous cords (**chordae tendineae**), which are in turn attached to small muscles located on the inner walls of the ventricles. These structures prevent inversion of the A-V valves under the high pressures created by the pumping action of the heart. The **semilunar valves** (aortic and pulmonary) are located at the roots of the **aorta** and the **pulmonary artery** respectively. These valves prevent a backflow of blood during the relaxation phase of the cardiac cycle.

Cardiac Vessels

The superior and inferior **venae cavae** return blood from the upper and lower extremities, respectively, to the right atrium. The pulmonary artery delivers blood from the right ventricle to the lungs, and **pulmonary veins** complete the circuit between the lungs and the left atrium. From the left ventricle, the aorta, the largest artery in the body, transports the blood through its branches to all parts of the body. It is important to understand that these vessels (except the aorta and the pulmonary artery) deliver blood to the chambers of the heart for pumping purposes only; none of this blood is actually used by the **myocardium** (heart muscle) as a source of oxygen. Oxygen and other nutrients necessary for myocardial function must come by way of the coronary arteries and their branches, which encircle and perfuse the myocardium.

Cardiac Innervation

The heart is capable of contraction independent of any extrinsic nerve supply. However, two external cardiac nerves are important. The **accelerator nerve,** which belongs to the sympathetic division of the autonomic nervous system, provides stimuli that increase heart rate. The **vagus nerve** presents stimuli from the parasympathetic division of the autonomic nervous system and serves to reduce heart rate.

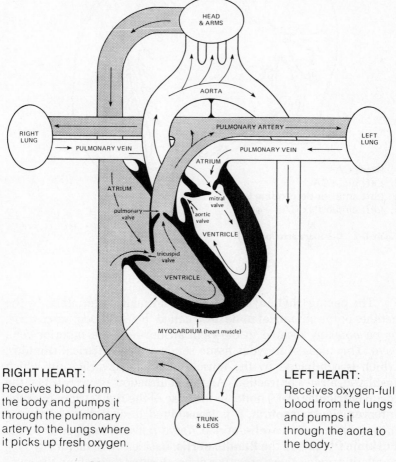

RIGHT HEART:
Receives blood from the body and pumps it through the pulmonary artery to the lungs where it picks up fresh oxygen.

LEFT HEART:
Receives oxygen-full blood from the lungs and pumps it through the aorta to the body.

Your Heart and How it Works

Figure 8-1. Your heart and how it works. (©American Heart Association. Reprinted with permission.)

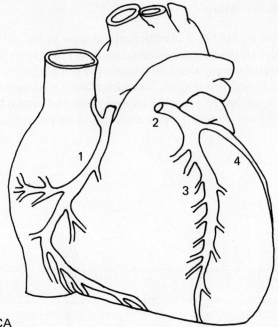

1. Right CA
2. Left main CA
3. Left anterior descending CA
4. Left circumflex CA

Figure 8-2. Coronary arteries (CA).

The pacing (rhythm) of the heart is normally determined by the activity of the **sinoatrial node** (also called the *S-A node, sinus node*, or *pacemaker*), located in the right atrium near the superior vena cava. This mass of nervous tissue sends out an electrical stimulus, which is conducted by the muscle cells of the atria, and which results in atrial contraction. As the contraction wave reaches the **atrioventricular (A-V) node,** in the base of the right atrium near the **interventricular septum,** it is transmitted through the ventricular myocardium over a well-defined nerve network composed of the **Purkinje fibers** and the **Bundle of His.** Besides these major rhythm-regulating nodes, there are other nodes, located throughout the myocardium, that can produce contraction in the event of a failure of the S-A or A-V nodes. Occasionally, one or more of these nodes becomes irritable and fires at random; this produces extra contractions, which are sometimes felt as extra beats or "skipped" beats. These are usually harmless but sometimes disturbing to the owner. In such cases, it is wise to consult a physician for accurate diagnosis. Equally important in such cases is the early establishment of an electrocardiographic base line, which can be helpful in the diagnosis of the relative severity or innocence of similar occurrences that might manifest themselves later. The reasons for these occasional innocent "short circuits" are not well understood. The increased nodal irritability that produces them is thought to be associated with cigarette smoking, use of drinks that contain caffeine, lack of rest, or stress.

CARDIAC CYCLE

In attempting to understand the relationship among the events of the cardiac cycle, one should be aware that the atria work as a unit, as do the ventricles; therefore, an occurrence on one side of the heart almost simultaneously takes place on the other side. It should also be understood that the right and left sides of the heart serve somewhat different functions. The right side receives deoxygenated blood (blood with a relatively high content of carbon dioxide and a somewhat reduced oxygen content) from the body, pumps it to the lungs to be oxygenated, and returns it to the left atrium. The left side receives this freshly oxygenated blood from the lungs via the pulmonary veins and pumps it to all parts of the body under enough pressure to ensure its return to the right atrium. Obviously, a much higher pressure must be generated by the left side of the heart—approximately five times as high as that developed by the right side—and, accordingly, the wall of the left side is much thicker and stronger.

The mechanical events that promote blood flow through the heart and the cardiovascular system can be classified in three categories, which characterize the three phases of the cardiac cycle. They are (1) **systole,** or contraction, (2) **diastole,** or relaxation, and (3) **diastasis,** or rest. These terms designate the state of the myocardial fibers at different times in the cycle. Each phase first occurs in the atria and then spreads to the ventricles. Although ventricular systole follows atrial systole very closely, the two do not occur simultaneously. The contracting, relaxing, and resting of the heart muscle, together with effective action of the valves, create pressure differentials between the chambers, which facilitate blood flow in the proper direction.

In describing the events of the cardiac cycle, one might begin at any point so long as the proper sequence is followed (e.g., diastole, diastasis, systole). Increases in heart rate decrease the amount of time allowed for a particular phase and can even eliminate diastasis completely; however, the normal sequence of events is unaffected.

Beginning with atrial diastasis, a simplified account of the most important events of the cardiac cycle follows: During atrial diastasis, the fibers encircling the atria are at rest, the A-V valves are open, and blood flows freely from the atria to the ventricles. At the onset of atrial systole, the stimulus from the pacemaker initiates contraction of the atrial fibers (atrial systole), which forces any blood that has collected in the atria into the ventricles. This ejection phase is followed by atrial diastole, at which time the atria are refilled. Even while the atria are contracting, the signal of the pacemaker is picked up by the A-V node and is distributed to the ventricular myocardium, which initiates ventricular systole. At the onset of this phase, the A-V valves, which were floated nearly closed during late diastole, are forcefully closed. The sound thus produced is fairly low-pitched and is caused, in part, by vibrations set up in the walls of the heart and the blood vessels by the closure of the valves. It is known as the *first heart sound*. Because the semilunar valves are also closed, ventricular blood is trapped. The pressure in the ventricles continues to build under increasing myocardial tension until it is greater than the pressure in the pulmonary artery and the aorta. At this time, the semilunar valves are forced open and the ventricles eject their blood. Immediately after ventricular systole, the fibers begin to relax, which marks the beginning of ventricular diastole. Pressure in the ventricle becomes lower than that in the aorta and the pulmonary artery, and the semilunar valves forcefully close. The sound thus created is the *second heart sound*; it is higher pitched and more crisp than the first. If a valve is structurally or functionally abnormal, additional sounds (**murmurs**) usually accompany the normal heart sounds [4, 5, 6]. (See Chapter 2.)

VASCULAR SYSTEM

To assist the heart in the delivery of blood throughout the body, three types of vessels are employed—arteries, veins, and capillaries. Functionally, the arteries carry blood away from the heart; the veins

TABLE 8-1
CHARACTERISTICS OF ARTERIES, VEINS, AND CAPILLARIES

Vessel	Diameter	Characteristics
Arteries	30 μ-2.5 cm	Walls thicker than those of corresponding veins Muscle tissue thicker than that in corresponding veins No apparent diffusion through walls
Veins	20 μ-3.0 cm	Walls thinner than those of corresponding arteries Muscle tissue thinner than that in corresponding arteries Valves present in larger veins No apparent diffusion through walls
Capillaries	1 μ-8 μ	Walls one cell thick, freely permit diffusion

return the blood to the heart; the capillaries are the connecting links between the arterial and venous trees, which allow respiratory gases and nutrients to be exchanged freely between the cells and the circulating blood. The duties of these vessels dictate that they be structurally different. Some of these differences are shown in Table 8-1.

CARDIOVASCULAR RESPONSES TO EXERCISE

Any discussion of cardiovascular responses to exercise must be qualified in terms of acute effects or long-term effects, because these types of responses are quite different. Furthermore, the kind of exercise employed is an important consideration. In this chapter, any reference to exercise or training should be taken to mean dynamic exercise (e.g., running or swimming) strenuous enough to elevate the heart rate to a sustained 140 to 150 beats per minute for at least 5 to 10 minutes.

To study circulatory responses to exercise, heart rate, blood pressure, stroke volume, and cardiac output are measured when the subject is at rest and again during submaximum and maximum exercise; comparisons are then made. It is generally accepted that the resting, untrained heart averages 70 to 80 beats per minute; however, these values may range from 50 to 90 beats per minute and still not indicate a pathologic condition. The typical heart rate of females is between 5 and 8 beats per minute higher than the typical rate for males. This may be because in females the heart is some-what smaller in relation to body size as is the stroke output per beat. If the average volume of blood ejected per stroke (70 to 80 milliliters) is multiplied by the average heart rate (70 to 80 beats per minute), the resulting output of the heart per minute (cardiac output) is approximately 4 to 6 liters of blood. The pressure generated by this outflow of blood against the artery walls is known as arterial blood pressure. Arterial pressure is pulsatile as is demonstrated by its elevation when the heart contracts and its fall when the heart relaxes. The peak resting pressure measured during contraction (systolic pressure) averages about 120 ± 20 millimeters of mercury. The pressure measured during relaxation of the ventricle (diastolic pressure) is lower; it averages about 80 ± 10 millimeters of mercury.

Acute Effects of Exercise

As an individual begins to exercise, the heart rate increases linearly in proportion to the severity of the work (see Figure 8-3). If

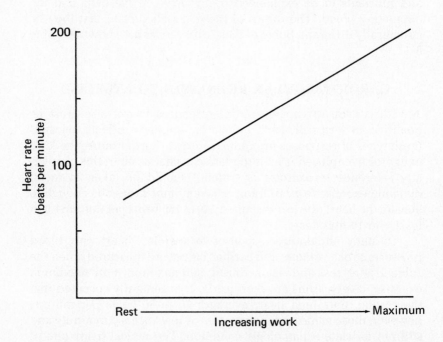

Figure 8-3. Heart rate response to increasing work loads.

the work is not maximal, the heart rate reaches a plateau after about 3 to 5 minutes and continues at that level for several minutes, again in proportion to the work load. This elevated heart rate is the result of an increased oxygen demand at the cellular level by the exercising muscles. The ultimate goal of the cardiovascular system is to increase cardiac output and thereby increase the delivery of blood to the areas that need it so that a balance between oxygen demanded and oxygen supplied can be achieved. This is accomplished by one or all of the following compensatory adjustments:

1. Increase in the heart rate
2. Increase in the stroke volume
3. Increase in the perfusion of the exercising tissue by means of flow through previously unopened capillaries
4. Increase in the amount of oxygen extracted from the blood by the working cells

Most people can elevate the effective heart rate to between two and three times the resting rate. In a majority of cases, the heart rate range (maximum rate minus resting rate) amounts to about 100 beats per minute, since 170 or 180 beats per minute is thought by many to be the greatest effective heart rate even though 200 and 210 beats per minute is not uncommon in individuals below age 20 [1].

The heart becomes a stronger pump due to the liberation of substances called *catecholamines*, which enable it to clear its ventricles more completely. As a result, stroke volume can be increased from 70 milliliters (when the individual is at rest) to almost double that amount (when a trained individual engages in heavy exercise).

In addition to these two adjustments, the capillary beds in the working muscles can open more completely to allow approximately three times more blood to enter; also *oxygen extraction* from a given volume of blood can be increased. Considering the combined effects of these adjustments, one can expect at least a 12-fold increase in the amount of blood delivered to the exercising tissue, in comparison with what is supplied during resting conditions.

During exercise, the systolic pressure in normal individuals increases linearly with the work load to a maximum value of about 240 millimeters of mercury. The normal diastolic-pressure response to physical effort is less predictable; it might increase or decrease slightly or remain unchanged. In trained persons, a slight decrease is usually observed as peripheral vascular resistance drops. In any case, an increase of more than 15 millimeters of mercury over the resting diastolic pressure is considered a hypertensive response.

It has been shown that arm work elicits higher blood pressures, ventilatory volumes, and heart rates than does work by the legs for an equivalent work load [3]. The significance of this finding applied to everyday life is that, because cardiovascular stress is greater during arm work, middle-aged, untrained individuals should be extremely cautious about sporadic heavy work with the arms (e.g., shoveling snow or soil, loading heavy items, or rowing). Furthermore, isometric work (straining against heavy resistance) should be discouraged, particularly in older people, because of the extremely high blood pressures and decreased venous return this type of activity produces.

REFERENCES

1. Astrand, P. O., and Rodahl, K. *Textbook of work physiology.* 2d ed. New York: McGraw-Hill, 1977.
2. Burton, A. C. *Physiology and biophysics of the circulation.* Chicago: Year Book Medical Publishers, 1965.
3. Clausen, J. P.; Trap-Jensen, J.; and Lassen, N. A. The effects of training in the heart rate during arm and leg exercise. *Scandinavian Journal of Clinical and Laboratory Investigation* 26:295–301, 1970.
4. Franklin, M.; Krauthhamer, M.; Tai, A. R.; and Pinchot, A. *The heart doctors' heart book.* New York: Bantam Books, 1976.
5. Guyton, A. C. *Textbook of medical physiology.* 5th ed. Philadelphia: W. B. Saunders, 1977.
6. Rushmer, R. F. *Cardiovascular dynamics.* Philadelphia: W. B. Saunders, 1970.

KEY TERMS
Aerobic capacity (p. 159)
Aerobic metabolism (p. 159)
Anaerobic metabolism (p. 160)
Maximum oxygen uptake (p. 158)
Oxygen debt (p. 160)
Pulmonary ventilation (p. 156)
Steady state (p. 160)

BEHAVIORAL OBJECTIVES
Upon completion of this chapter, the student
should be able to:
1. Define the key terms listed above.
2. Describe the mechanism of oxygen delivery
   to the cells.
3. Identify the adjustments the respiratory system makes during exercise.
4. Demonstrate the role of dead space air in
   reducing alveolar ventilation.

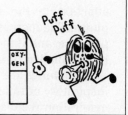

It is unrealistic to discuss the role of the circulatory system in exercise and training without a treatment of the contributions of the respiratory system as well. In fact, increasing one's ability to deliver blood to working tissue is quite futile without a concomitant improvement in the respiratory system. Fortunately, the two systems are related so that activities that develop one also stimulate improvement in the other. Therefore, many writers combine the systems and speak of the *circulorespiratory (CR) system.*

BASIC COMPONENTS OF THE RESPIRATORY SYSTEM

The basic components of the respiratory system are as follows:
1. Entryways (mouth and nose)
2. Trachea (windpipe)
3. Primary bronchi
4. Lungs (composed of many branches of *bronchioles* that through about 23 sets of subdivisions finally terminate in a *respiratory bronchiole* with its alveolar sacs)

Figure 9-1 shows these structures along with several important surrounding structures that enclose the lung in the thoracic cavity and that assist breathing. The reader should understand that the exchange of oxygen and carbon dioxide in the lung takes place in the alveoli only. The air between the entryways and the alveoli is not involved in any exchange.

MECHANICS OF BREATHING

Breathing, also called **pulmonary ventilation,** consists of inhaling air (that contains among other things 21% oxygen and 0.04% carbon dioxide) and exhaling lung air (14.2% oxygen and 5.5% carbon dioxide). At rest, inspiration is actively assisted by muscular contraction, whereas expiration is passive. The mechanics of the system require that inspiration occur when the *intercostal muscles* and the *diaphragm* contract. This causes the size of the thoracic cavity to increase, and therefore the lungs also expand because they are attached to the wall of the thoracic cavity by means of the pleura.The increase in volume results in a decrease in intrathoracic pressure, and if the passages to the lungs are unobstructed, air flows in to equalize the pressure.

The lungs are elastic and are stretched by the contraction of the inspiratory muscles. Consequently, the relaxation of the muscles of inspiration results in diminished thoracic size and elastic recoil of

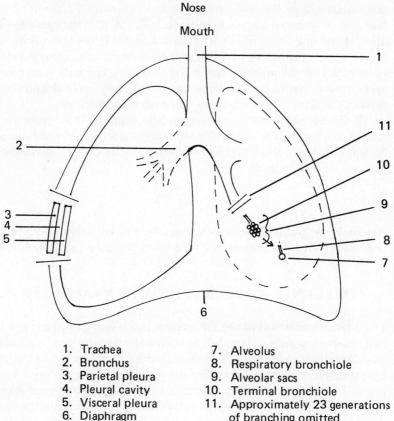

Figure 9-1. The lung.

1. Trachea
2. Bronchus
3. Parietal pleura
4. Pleural cavity
5. Visceral pleura
6. Diaphragm

7. Alveolus
8. Respiratory bronchiole
9. Alveolar sacs
10. Terminal bronchiole
11. Approximately 23 generations
    of branching omitted

the lung tissue, which increases intrathoracic pressure and drives air out of the lungs. During exercise, however, when the lungs need to be emptied more rapidly or more completely than during rest, additional muscles are brought into play [1, 3].

LUNG VOLUMES

A normal adult lung holds maximally about 6,200 to 7,400 milliliters of air. The actual amount depends upon specific body dimensions. However, about 1,200 milliliters of maximum lung capacity (*residual air*) are never expelled. This means that the maximum amount of air

air) is never expelled. This means that the maximum amount of air that can be expired after a maximum inspiration (*vital capacity*) is about 4,500 to 6,000 milliliters for men and 3,000 to 4,500 milliliters for women. During normal breathing while at rest, only a small portion (about 500 milliliters) of maximum lung capacity is inspired and expired (exchanged) during one respiratory cycle (inspiration plus expiration). This amount is referred to as *tidal air.*

If the normal respiratory frequency is assumed to be between 8 and 18 respiratory cycles per minute and the average tidal volume to be 500 milliliters, it is quite easy to calculate the *minute ventilatory volume* by the formula

$$\dot{V}_E = V_T \times f$$

where $\dot{V}_E$ = pulmonary ventilation, V_T = tidal volume (depth of breathing), and f = respiratory frequency (breaths per minute) [4].

OXYGEN AND CARBON DIOXIDE TRANSPORT

The primary function of the CR system is the delivery of oxygen to cells in the quantity demanded by metabolic activity at a particular site. Equally important is the removal of carbon dioxide and other by-products of metabolism. The hemoglobin in circulating blood plays the major role in this oxygen/carbon dioxide transport function. As a result of differences in pressure of oxygen and carbon dioxide in the lungs and pulmonary capillaries and at the cellular level, diffusion gradients are established. These gradients, whose effects are enhanced by the affinity of hemoglobin for the two gases, facilitate its loading with oxygen and unloading of carbon dioxide in the capillaries of the lung and its unloading of oxygen and loading with carbon dioxide at the cellular level.

Under normal conditions of health and at normal atmospheric pressure, blood is about 98% saturated with oxygen when it leaves the lung. In a resting person, about 30% of this oxygen is removed at the cellular level, but during heavy exercise, this amount can be increased almost three times. The amount of oxygen extracted from circulating blood in 1 minute is termed *oxygen uptake.* If measured during maximum exercise, this quantity is **maximum oxygen uptake,** which is believed by exercise physiologists to be the best single indicator of physical fitness because it represents the ability of the body to mobilize all its systems during physical stress.

OXYGEN REQUIREMENT

Oxygen consumption ($\dot{V}O_2$) in an individual at rest is about 0.25 liters/min, or about 3.5 ml/kg of body weight per minute. During heavy exercise, this value can be increased 12 to 16 times depending on the relative state of CR fitness. The maximum $\dot{V}O_2$ that one can attain (**aerobic capacity**) measures the effectiveness of the heart, lungs, and vascular system in the delivery of oxygen during heavy work—the higher the $\dot{V}O_2$ max, the more effective the system.

Values for $\dot{V}O_2$ are usually reported in liters per minute. However, when comparisons between individuals are made or when classification into a fitness category is desired, adjustments must be made for body size. This is achieved by dividing the $\dot{V}O_2$ in liters per minute by the body weight in kilograms. The resulting value is expressed in milliliters of O_2 consumed per kilogram of body weight per minute of work.

Oxygen uptake in untrained young males generally ranges from 42 to 45 ml/kg of body weight per minute of work. Values for females are 3 to 4 milliliters lower at the same level of fitness. With proper training this value may be elevated to range from 50 to 55 ml/kg of body weight per minute, which is considered to indicate excellent CR fitness. Although many endurance athletes have been able to achieve oxygen uptakes as high as 65 to 70 ml/kg of body weight per minute, a few biologically gifted individuals have been able to combine their hereditary traits with very hard training to develop capacities for processing more than 70 ml O_2/kg of body weight per minute. This last group describes the elite few who become world class champions in endurance events. Frank Shorter, an Olympic marathon gold medalist, and Bill Rodgers, three-time winner of the Boston Marathon, with 71 and 78 ml/kg of body weight per minute, respectively, are examples of athletes in this category.

OXYGEN DEBT

For cellular metabolism to continue for very long, adequate oxygen must be supplied (**aerobic metabolism**). This is not always possible, however. Two examples in which the supply is inadequate occur (1) at the beginning of heavy work, when the oxygen demand is greater than the response capability of the transport system, and (2) during heavy work at a very high intensity, when the oxygen demand is greater than the transport capacity of the cardiovascular system. In either case, the body is capable of working for short periods because of a process called **anaerobic metabolism.** When muscles operate anaerobically, an **oxygen debt** is created and must be repaid at a later time. Small oxygen debts are formed each time one deviates appreciably from the resting state, but these are rapidly repaid when the exercise ceases, because little or no *lactic acid* (a by-product of anaerobic metabolism) accumulates.

During work that requires less than 50% of one's aerobic capacity, the oxygen transport system is usually able to supply adequate amounts of oxygen to working tissue. When this happens, heart rate, ventilation, and $\dot{V}O_2$ can be maintained at a constant level for indefinite periods of time. This constitutes a balance between supply and demand and is termed **steady state.**

If, however, one engages in work that demands more than 50% of the aerobic capacity, the oxygen transport system is unable to supply as much as is demanded, and an oxygen debt is created. Anaerobic pathways of energy production are called into play so that the individual can continue working. This allows continued short-term performance, although working time is significantly reduced as lactic acid rapidly builds up. When the oxygen debt reaches about 15 liters, work must cease to allow for repayment and removal of some of the metabolic wastes that accumulated during the anaerobic work.

RECOVERY AFTER EXERCISE

One is fully recovered after exercise only when blood pressure, heart rate, ventilation, and $\dot{V}O_2$ have returned to preexercise levels. The amount of time required for recovery is a function of the intensity and the duration of the exercise and the relative state of training of the individual. One recovers faster if the oxygen debt incurred during the exercise is a moderate one in which the *lactacid* component is very small.

RESPIRATORY PHENOMENA

Several interesting respiratory phenomena appear from time to time in some individuals and deserve mention.

Second Wind

During the early minutes of vigorous work, uncomfortably difficult breathing (dyspnea) may occur. In some individuals, accompanying characteristics such as dizziness, heavy legs, chest pain, and general physical discomfort are also reported. However, after a few minutes of continuous work at the same intensity, these symptoms seem to disappear, the distress subsides, and one experiences a "second wind." This phenomenon is more common in untrained persons than in well-trained athletes, or in those who have not warmed up properly. The explanation is related to the fact that the circulorespiratory system does not become fully efficient for 3 to 5 minutes of work at a moderate intensity. During this time lag, metabolic wastes accumulate. When full efficiency is achieved, the distress subsides somewhat as a result of improved oxygen delivery to working muscles and removal of the waste products of anaerobic metabolism.

Side Stitch

A side stitch often develops in untrained persons during running activities. This is evident as a sharp pain in the area of the lower rib cage and is usually confined to the right side of the body. Several explanations have been offered, none of which is completely satisfactory. It is probable that all of the following factors contribute to the discomfort:

1. Accumulation of metabolic wastes (lactic acid) in the diaphragm
2. Severe shaking of the abdominal contents, which causes pain in the supporting structures
3. Formation of gas in the ascending colon
4. Reduced blood flow to the affected area due to the rerouting of blood to other areas

As with second wind, side stitch rarely occurs in trained individuals. Relief is hastened by the application of pressure on the affected side while the exercise is continued. If the pain becomes too severe, the only alternative is to terminate the work.

VENTILATION DURING RUNNING

Runners are often concerned about the efficiency of their methods of ventilating the lungs during exercise. They wonder whether they should breathe faster as the demands of exercise increase or whether they should breathe deeper. While the answer is not clear for all levels of exercise, some insight into the problem might be gained from the following example.

Assume that a runner at rest is breathing at a rate (f) of 10 times per minute and at a depth (V_T) of 0.5 liter per breath. From the ventilation equation found on page 158, it can be seen that the pulmonary ventilation ($\dot{V}_E$) is 5.0 liters/min.

$$\dot{V}_E = V_T \times f$$
$$= 0.5 \text{ liter/breath} \times 10 \text{ breaths/min}$$
$$= 5.0 \text{ liter/min}$$

Suppose that, during exercise, the runner's ventilatory demand increases to 20 liters/min. The question is whether the demand should be satisfied by an increase in tidal volume or in rate, or both. At this low level, the answer clearly favors an increase in the depth if the runner's desire is to remain efficient. The reason concerns repeated movement of dead space air (DSA) and can be explained as follows:

Although pulmonary ventilation describes the air flow to and from the lungs, alveolar ventilation ($\dot{V}_A$) represents the portion of pulmonary ventilation that actually reaches the alveolar level to participate in the oxygen/carbon dioxide exchange with pulmonary capillary blood. DSA is the volume of air that is contained in the respiratory passageways. Because it amounts roughly to 1 ml/lb of body weight, this volume is estimated to be 150 milliliters for the so-called "average man." DSA might be considered stagnant because it never reaches the alveoli nor is it completely flushed out during expiration. Consequently, it does not contribute to effective ventilation of the alveoli. Its volume must be deducted from the tidal volume per breath to arrive at a value for alveolar ventilation [2]. In terms of the preceding example, the runner's ventilatory requirement of 20 liters/min could be satisfied, on the one hand, by an increase in rate alone as follows:

$$\dot{V}_E = V_T \times f$$
$$= 0.500 \times 40 = 20 \text{ liters/min}$$

$$\dot{V}_A = (V_T - DSA) \times f$$
$$= (0.500 - 0.150) \times 40$$
$$= 0.350 \times 40$$
$$= 14 \text{ liters/min}$$

On the other hand, the requirement could be met by an increase in tidal volume alone:

$$\dot{V}_E = V_T \times f$$
$$= 2.000 \times 10 = 20 \text{ liters/min}$$

$$\dot{V}_A = (V_T - DSA) \times f$$
$$= (2.000 - 0.150) \times 10$$
$$= 1.850 \times 10$$
$$= 18.5 \text{ liters/min}$$

From this example, it should be clear that alveolar ventilation is enhanced more by an increase in tidal volume than by an increase in frequency. While this holds true for most submaximum levels of work, there is a point at which the metabolic cost of deep breathing outweighs its advantage. At any rate, it appears helpful to consciously attempt to increase tidal volume to satisfy greater ventilatory demands during submaximum work. Many distance runners advocate that this increase in tidal volume be accomplished by "belly breathing," which they claim is more efficient than intercostal (chest) breathing.

REFERENCES

1. Astrand, P. O., and Rodahl, K. *Textbook of work physiology*. 2d ed. New York: McGraw-Hill, 1977.
2. Comroe, J. H. *Physiology of respiration*. Chicago: Yearbook Medical Publishers, 1965.
3. Guyton, A. C. *Textbook of medical physiology*. 5th ed. Philadelphia: W. B. Saunders, 1977.
4. Slonim, N. B., and Hamilton, L. H. *Respiratory physiology*. 2d ed. St. Louis: C. V. Mosby, 1971.

KEY TERMS
All-or-none law (p. 166)
Body alignment (p. 174)
Center of gravity (p. 171)
Force application (p. 173)
Force arm (p. 174)
Kinesthetic perception (p. 171)
Motor unit (p. 169)
Muscle fiber (p. 166)
Myofibrils (p. 167)
Posture (p. 174)
Resistance application (p. 173)
Resistance arm (p. 174)
Sarcolemma (p. 167)
Sarcoplasm (p. 167)
Stability (p. 171)

BEHAVIORAL OBJECTIVES
Upon completion of this chapter, the student should be able to:

1. Define the key terms listed above.
2. Describe the characteristics of skeletal, smooth, and cardiac muscle tissue.
3. Identify and describe the components of the gross structure of skeletal muscle.
4. Diagram a skeletal muscle fiber; label and define the sarcomere, actin, and myosin filaments, Z-line, H-zone, A-band, and I-band.
5. Describe the sliding-filament theory and the role of adenosine triphosphate (ATP).
6. Identify the factors responsible for gradation of muscular contraction.
7. List and define the types of muscular contraction.
8. Define the principles of reciprocal innervation, equilibrium, and levers; describe the relationship and importance of these principles to movement skills.
9. Describe the three classes of levers; state one mechanical example for each class and one anatomical example for first-class and third-class levers.
10. Describe good posture and movement mechanics for standing, walking, running for speed, running for distance, sitting, lifting, carrying heavy objects, and lying.

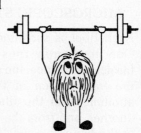

People cannot do anything without using some muscle, or muscles, as all movement and body functions depend upon the contraction of muscle tissue. There are three types of muscle tissue in the human body—skeletal, smooth and cardiac.

Skeletal, striated muscle performs the functions of moving and stabilizing the skeletal system. It is innervated by the voluntary (somatic) nervous system and consists of long, cylindrical **muscle fibers.** Each fiber, or cell, has several hundred nuclei and is structurally independent of other fibers. Skeletal muscle is called *striated* because of its parallel layers of alternating light and dark bands.

Smooth, nonstriated muscle is found in the walls of the hollow organs and blood vessels. It is innervated by the involuntary (autonomic) nervous system and ordinarily is not under voluntary control. Smooth muscle consists of long, spindle-shaped cells, and each cell usually has only one nucleus.

Cardiac muscle, the heart muscle, is a network of striated fibers. The arrangment of the fibers enables the cardiac muscle to contract as a unit, obeying the **all-or-none law.** Cardiac muscle also contracts rhythmically and automatically because the impulse for contraction originates within the heart itself.

GROSS STRUCTURE OF SKELETAL MUSCLE

Skeletal muscle has an outside covering of connective tissue called the *epimysium,* which merges with a tendon at the ends of the muscle. The tendon connects the muscle to a bone.

Within a muscle, the fibers are grouped into bundles, referred to as *fasciculi* (fasciculus is singular), which are covered by a connective tissue called the *perimysium.* The fasciculi vary in length and ordinarily do not run the full length of a large muscle. A fasciculus may have only a few muscle fibers or as many as 150 or more. (See Figure 10-1.)

MICROSCOPIC STRUCTURE OF SKELETAL MUSCLE

Each fiber is surrounded by connective tissue, the *endomysium.* One fiber rarely runs the entire length of a muscle or even of a fasciculus. Hence, the connective tissue of a muscle is necessary for the transmission of the force of contraction from one fiber to another, from the fibers to a fasciculus, from one fasciculus to another, and from the fasciculi to the tendon or tendons connected to the bone.

The smallest fibers cannot be seen with the naked eye, and the largest are as thick as a human hair. They range in length from 1 to 50 mm, which in some cases is the entire length of the muscle.

Beneath the endomysium, the muscle cell is covered by a tough, exceedingly thin, elastic sheath, the **sarcolemma,** and beneath it are located the numerous nuclei. Embedded in the muscle-fiber protoplasm (**sarcoplasm**) are columnlike structures called **myofibrils.** (It is the myofibrils, with alternating segments of light and dark, that provide the striated appearance of skeletal muscle.) Each myofibril is subdivided into *sarcomeres.* These are the functional units of the myofibrils and are composed of two types of parallel, proteinaceous filaments: thick filaments containing *myosin* and thin ones containing *actin.*

As shown in Figure 10-2, the thin filaments of actin form a light zone called the *I-band,* and the thick myosin filaments form the denser, darker *A-band.* The actin filaments arise from a membrane called the *Z-line,* which forms the boundary between the sarcomeres. The spaces between pairs of actin filaments form a lighter band within the A-band, called the *H-zone.*

THE CONTRACTILE PROCESS

The most widely accepted explanation of muscle contraction is the *sliding-filament theory.* It contends that the actin filaments slide

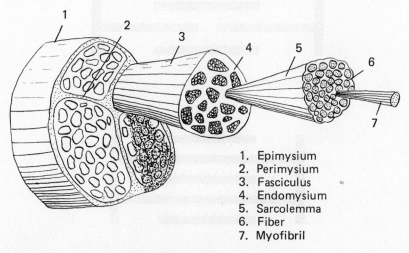

1. Epimysium
2. Perimysium
3. Fasciculus
4. Endomysium
5. Sarcolemma
6. Fiber
7. Myofibril

Figure 10-1. Construction of a skeletal muscle.

between the myosin filaments, which pulls the Z-lines of the sarcomere toward the A-band and shortens the I-band. The length of the A-band is not changed; that is, the myosin filaments remain constant in length. However, the H-zone disappears in the sliding process. (See Figure 10-2.) The exact manner in which this process occurs is not completely understood, but it is believed that cross-bridges from the myosin filaments form a chemical bond with selected sites on the actin filaments.

Energy for muscle contraction is derived from the breakdown of *adenosine triphosphate (ATP)*. Nerve impulses sent to the muscle cell stimulate this breakdown, and the energy yielded is used when the actin filaments slide between the myosin filaments. The liberation of energy occurs in the following reaction: ATP → *adenosine*

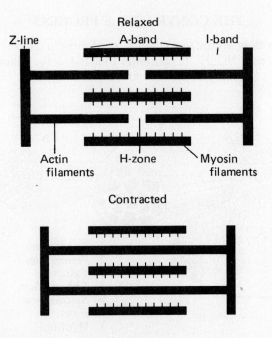

Figure 10-2. Structure of a sarcomere.

diphosphate (ADP) + phosphate + energy. ATP for further contraction is synthesized from nutrient substances and creatine phosphate. The latter, which is found only in muscle tissue, is broken down by enzymes during exercise; its by-products combine with ADP to form ATP:

$$\text{creatine phosphate} \xrightarrow{\text{enzyme}} \text{creatine} + \text{phosphates} + \text{energy}$$

$$\text{phosphates} + \text{energy} + \text{ADP} \rightleftarrows \text{ATP}$$

THE MOTOR UNIT

The basic unit of muscular contraction is the **motor unit**, which consists of a group of muscle cells innervated by the fiber of a single nerve cell. Upon entering the muscle through the epimysium, the nerve fiber branches and distributes itself among the muscle cells. The need for this arrangement can be seen in the huge difference that exists between the number of *motor nerves* entering a muscle and the number of muscle fibers (cells) within the muscle: there are about 250,000,000 separate muscle fibers that make up the human skeletal muscles, but there are only approximately 420,000 motor nerves [4]. As every muscle fiber must be innervated, it is necessary that nerve fibers branch repeatedly.

The number of muscle fibers in a motor unit varies from muscle to muscle in relation to the function of the muscle. Muscles performing fine and delicate work, such as those of the eye, may have ratios of one nerve fiber to five or fewer muscle fibers, whereas muscles used for heavy work may have 150 or more muscle fibers per motor unit.

THE ALL-OR-NONE LAW

A muscle rarely contracts to its maximum as an entire unit, but a single fiber can only contract maximally. Upon receiving a nerve impulse that is strong enough to cause contraction, an individual muscle fiber either contracts completely or does not contract at all. Because a single nerve cell supplies all the muscle fibers of a motor unit, the motor unit also follows the all-or-none law.

The contraction force of the entire muscle varies in relation to a given set of conditions at the time of contraction. If appropriate nutrients are available and the muscle is warm and is not fatigued, the contraction can be strong. However, a weak contraction results if the muscle is cold and fatigued and the needed nutrients are not present.

MUSCLE FATIGUE

Fatigue occurs when the contractile and metabolic processes of muscle fibers are no longer able to maintain an established work rate. Exercise physiologists do not agree upon what is the site of muscular fatigue. Its causes may include changes in the chemical properties of the muscle fibers, breakdown of the ATP/ADP system, depletion of the glycogen stores, and inability to remove the end products that accumulate during anaerobic work.

GRADATION OF MUSCULAR CONTRACTION

The strength, or gradation, of contraction is determined not by the individual motor unit but by two other factors. One is the number of motor units stimulated. A muscle might contain hundreds of motor units and, although all the fibers of a single motor unit must contract together, the many motor units of one muscle do not have to contract at the same time. The size of the work load is evaluated by the brain and it stimulates an appropriate number of motor units. Sometimes an incorrect judgment is made, and more motor units are stimulated than are needed, as happens when one lifts an empty box that was believed to contain a heavy load. Conversely, too few motor units are stimulated when one first lifts a heavy box that was believed to be light.

The second factor in the gradation of muscular response is the frequency of stimulation, or the number of times per second that each motor unit is stimulated. If the muscle fibers are stimulated a second time before they relax from the first contraction, a second contraction will be added to the first. The total response to the two stimuli which are close together is larger than the response to a single stimulus.

TYPES OF CONTRACTION

Muscular contraction can result in shortening, maintaining a static position, or lengthening. Examples of these types of contraction follow.

During *isotonic contraction,* the muscle changes in length while a constant tension is applied to it. Shortening of the sarcomeres and movement take place. Push-ups, work with weights, and sit-ups require this type of contraction. *Dynamic* and *concentric contraction* are other names for isotonic contraction.

If a muscle remains a constant length during contraction, *isometric,* or *static, contraction* takes place. Pushing and pulling against an immovable object produce isometric contraction.

The gradual lengthening of a muscle from a shortened position is *eccentric contraction.* The triceps undergo eccentric contraction when they return to the down position during push-ups, as do the biceps brachii when the body is slowly lowered during chin-ups.

All three types of contraction have been used to increase strength; however, each has recognized advantages and disadvantages. Training regimens employing these types of contraction are discussed in greater detail in Chapter 4.

MECHANICAL PRINCIPLES

At rest or in motion, people must apply certain mechanical principles if general efficiency, reduction of energy expenditure, and improvement of physical performance are to take place. Of these mechanical principles reciprocal innervation, equilibrium, and levers will be discussed.

Reciprocal Innervation

For coordinated and graceful movement to occur, the muscles opposite the contracting muscles must be able to relax and lengthen easily. All muscles must also be able to contract strongly and quickly [5].

The ability to feel this contraction and relaxation, to know what a muscle is doing, to know the position of body parts, is **kinesthetic perception.** A person who fails to develop this ability has no basis for feeling and sensing whether a movement is right or wrong and no basis for correcting an error in movement or for establishing a movement pattern. Kinesthetic perception develops as one consciously places the body or its parts in a position and "gets the feel" of that position. With practice, this ability to feel becomes habitual and serves as an important force for increasing the efficiency of movement [5].

Equilibrium

Equilibrium involves balance, **stability,** position, and stance. There can be various stages of stability and the **center of gravity** is involved in all of them. The center of gravity is the weight center of a body, the imaginary point at which all the body's parts exactly balance one another. For the human body, its location depends upon the individual's structure, posture, and position. If a person of average build stands erect with the arms hanging at the sides, the center of gravity is located in the pelvis, in front of the upper sacrum. A woman's center of gravity is usually lower than a man's because of her heavier pelvis and thighs and her shorter legs. The center of gravity can be shifted by a change in posture or a movement of the limbs and also by external weights that the body supports.

The ability to maintain stability is affected by all of the following factors [3].

1. The wider the body's base of support, the greater the stability. An individual standing erect with the feet spread about 12 to 14 inches apart is in a more stable position than one who stands with the feet very close together. Positions that place both hands and knees or feet on the ground establish a wider base and hence greater stability.

2. Stability is decreased as the center of gravity moves horizontally closer to the edge of the support base. A sprinter on the starting line leans forward so that the center of gravity is directly above the hands. This position creates a tendency to fall forward, which enables the runner to start quicker than someone whose center of gravity is over the feet.

3. The heavier the body's weight, the greater the stability. If two individuals assume postures with the same base of support, it is more difficult to move the heavier individual.

4. If the base of support remains the same width, stability is decreased as the center of gravity moves higher. The closer the center of gravity to the base of support, the greater the stability.

5. For equilibrium to exist, a vertical line through the body's center of gravity must fall within the base of support. If the center of gravity moves outside the base, the individual becomes less stable and more likely to fall. To perform a handstand, for example, the individual must maintain the center of gravity directly over the area between the hands.

Principles of Levers

A lever is a rigid bar that turns about a fixed point or an axis by the application of an external force. The purpose of a lever is to gain mechanical advantage, so that a small force can overcome a larger

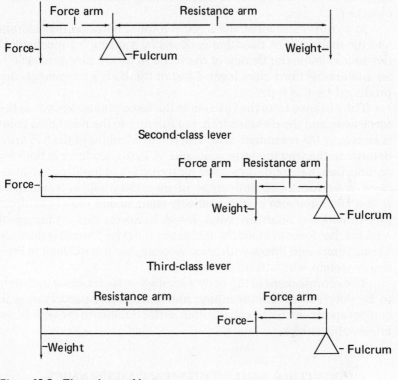

Figure 10-3. Three classes of levers.

resistance. In the body, the bones serve as levers, and muscle contractions produce the forces that operate them. The resistances to motion can be internal or external or both [6].

The classification and effectiveness of a lever is dependent upon the location of three points: the fulcrum (axis), the point of **force application**, and the point of **resistance application** (see Figure 10-3). If the fulcrum is located between the force and the resistance, it is designated a *first-class lever,* which is the most efficient kind. A teeter board and scissors are mechanical first-class levers; the extension of the forearm by the triceps muscle and the flexion and extension of the head are anatomical first-class levers.

If the resistance is located between the fulcrum and the force, it is designated a *second-class lever.* A wheelbarrow is one example.

Whether or not there are any second-class levers in the body appears to be a controversial matter among anatomists and kinesi-ologists [7].

In a *third-class lever,* the force is located between the fulcrum and the resistance. A door that is closed by a spring is a mechanical third-class lever; the flexion of the forearm by the biceps muscle is an anatomical third-class lever. Most of the body's movements are produced by this type.

The distance from the fulcrum to the force point is known as the **force arm,** and the distance from the fulcrum to the resistance point is known as the **resistance arm.** The relative lengths of the two arms determine the way the lever functions. A first-class lever is built for equilibrium, a second-class lever for reduction of force, and a third-class lever for speed and range of movement [6]. In anatomical levers, the force arm is comparatively short so that muscle contraction provides a relatively weak force; however, this arrangement enables that force to move the resistance quickly. Thus, it is possible to run, jump, and throw with great velocity, but it is difficult to lift a heavy weight with a third-class lever.

The arrangement of the body's leverage system causes the joints to be very susceptible to injury, and individuals participating in contact sports, such as football, often suffer damage to the shoulders, knees, and ankles.

POSTURE AND MOVEMENT MECHANICS

For efficient movement to take place, correct **posture (body align-ment)** is mandatory. The postures that are maintained for various positions and movements are the result of conscious and uncon-scious practice, which usually leads to the formation of postural habits. They may be good habits, which contribute to attractive appearance and to mechanical efficiency, or they may be poor habits, which contribute to incorrect muscle development, tension, spinal deviations, lower back disorders, poor circulation, and unat-tractive appearance.

Postural habits are developed as a person repeatedly assumes a given body alignment during work, play, and relaxation. While one is in this position, a response is established in the neuromuscular system. This response becomes habitual so that it is produced even though the individual is unconscious of posture. The habitual pos-tural response occurs whether the habit is good or bad, and many individuals mistakenly feel comfortable in a position that actually places a strain on the joints [5].

The habits of poor posture cannot be overcome with a few minutes of daily exercise. The neuromuscular system must be given thorough reeducation over an extended period to establish good body alignment and mechanics.

In summary, Metheny [5] describes the following conditions as fundamental for the development of effective posture and movement: (1) every muscle should have sufficient strength and tone to perform its functions; (2) every muscle should have sufficient relaxation to perform its functions easily; (3) the joints should have flexibility that provides for a full range of movement; (4) kinesthetic perception should be highly developed; and (5) good posture development should be continuous throughout the day and should be controlled to produce the best results in strength, relaxation, flexibility, and efficiency of movement.

These conditions can be met by a person who has (1) a knowledge of the movement process and the mechanics of efficient movement, (2) the ability to control his or her neuromuscular system, and (3) the desire to acquire an effective posture [5]. The following mechanical descriptions provide the knowledge necessary for an individual to experience efficient posture and movement.

Standing [8]

1. The head and chin are centered over the trunk and are held in a relaxed position at right angles to the front of the neck.
2. The shoulders are free and easy and are neither forward, back, nor elevated.
3. The shoulder blades are drawn down and flat on the back.
4. The chest is held up and is neither sagging nor too high nor leading.
5. The trunk is within normal limits of curves, neither too straight and flat nor too round and hollow.
6. The abdomen is up and in and is neither relaxed nor protruding.
7. The hips are in line with the trunk and are neither leading nor thrust back.
8. The arms hang naturally and relaxed at the sides and are neither held rigidly nor too relaxed.
9. The knees are free and easy and are neither bent nor thrust back.
10. The feet are parallel and slightly apart.

11. The weight falls ahead of the outer anklebone and is distributed toward the outside of each foot.

From the front view of this position, the weight should be evenly distributed about a vertical line through the midpoint of the body. From the side view, a vertical line should pass through the earlobe, through the middle of the shoulder and the middle of the hip, slightly behind the kneecap, and slightly in front of the outer anklebone. The center of gravity should be directly over the base of support.

Walking [5]

1. The upper body (head, chin, shoulders, and chest) should be balanced on the trunk; it should not be dragged forward by the pull of gravity.
2. The trunk should be balanced in the pelvic basin; it does not come to an erect, rigid position between steps, but remains inclined slightly forward to keep it in line with the extended rear leg at the time of the push-off. The center of gravity should not be carried beyond the base of support.
3. Motion should originate in the hip joint as the leading leg is swung ahead of the body.
4. The leading leg is always parallel to or in advance of the trunk so that a new base of support is always ready to receive the body weight.
5. As a new base of support is established, the upper body remains in line with the axis of the rear leg.
6. The supporting and pushing leg applies its force directly through the center of gravity along the line of resistance of the trunk. This leg begins to push off before the front foot strikes the ground.
7. The heel strikes the ground first, directly in line with the direction of walk. The weight is transferred through the outer border of the foot to the ball of the foot.
8. The ankle joint is extended as the final push or thrust is made with the big toe.
9. The weight shift to the alternate foot causes the pelvic girdle to oscillate back and forth. The arms and shoulders swing slightly to compensate for this oscillation and to keep the body weight evenly distributed.
10. The leg muscles should supply most of the energy for locomotion so that the body makes as few extraneous motions as possible.

Running for Speed [2, 3]

1. The trunk should be upright to keep the runner in balance. Leaning forward places the body off balance, which forces the leg muscles to exert additional effort to prevent a fall. With the trunk upright, the center of gravity can be forward of the pushing foot.
2. Because a long lever develops more speed at the end than does a short lever, the lead leg should be fully extended at the moment of the push from the rear leg. This action also enables the full force of the push to be converted into forward movement.
3. Any vertical movement should be just great enough to counteract the downward pull of gravity but not great enough to produce an unnecessary bounce, because the forward speed of the runner is decreasing while the body is off the ground. The higher the center of gravity rises, the longer the body is off the ground.
4. As the foot leaves the ground after a vigorous push, the knee is bent. The faster the leg moves, the more the knee is bent, and the higher the foot is raised. By this action, the knee moves forward with greater angular velocity owing to the shorter radius of the arc through which the leg swings.
5. The faster one moves, the higher the knee should be raised in front. This movement delays the placing of the foot on the ground for its next thrust and permits the lead leg to reach full extension.
6. The runner should alight on the ball of the foot.
7. The faster one runs, the longer the stride. However, if the stride is too long, the runner's foot contacts the ground ahead of the center of gravity, which produces a braking action.
8. The swing of the arms should be coordinated with that of the legs in order to balance the rotary effect of the leg swing on the trunk.

Running for Distance [1]

1. The head should remain up to avoid the tendency to watch the feet.
2. The back should be straight but naturally comfortable. Do not throw back the shoulders and stick out the chest.
3. The buttocks should be tucked in. In this position, a hypothetical line drawn through the shoulders and the hips should be vertical or nearly so.

4. The elbows are bent and held slightly away from the body. One should avoid placing them out like wings or pressing them to the chest; they should be carried slightly above hip or belt level.
5. The body should be straight as the legs move freely from the hips. The legs should be lifted from the knees while the ankles are relaxed. The runner should not overstride; each foot should fall just under the knee.
6. Using the heel-to-toe method for footstrike, one should land on the heel, then rock forward to take off from the ball of the foot. This method is the least tiring over long distances and is the least wearing because the heel cushions the landing and the forward rocking distributes the pressure.
7. In the flat-foot method for footstrike, the foot falls under the knee in a quick, light action with the entire foot landing on the ground at the same time. This type of landing provides a wide surface area to cushion the footstrike. The foot should not be driven down but should be allowed to pass beneath the body.

Sitting [5]

1. The head, neck, and shoulders should be in the same position as for standing.
2. The back of the buttocks should touch the back of the chair. All the support of the chair should be used.
3. The feet should be flat on the floor. There may be variations in the position of the legs and feet, but the hips should remain toward the back of the chair.
4. If one writes or reads while sitting at a table, the chair should be brought well under the table, so that the edge of the table almost touches the front of the body. Sit all the way back in the chair and allow the trunk to slant forward slightly from the hip joint to bring the eyes in line with the work. Keep the head-neck-trunk line as straight as possible for maximum support of the head.

Lifting Heavy Objects

1. The knees should be bent and the back should remain straight.
2. The feet should be spread apart about shoulder width.
3. The lifting should be performed by straightening the legs.

Carrying Heavy Objects

1. The center of gravity should always be above the base of support.
2. The body alignment should be altered as little as possible.

3. The object should be carried as close to the body's center of gravity as possible and no higher than waist level.

Lying

1. If one is lying on the back, a pillow should be placed under the knees to help prevent exaggerated curvature of the lower back. The head should be elevated only slightly.
2. If one is lying on the side, both knees should be drawn up to relieve lower back strain.
3. If one is lying on the stomach, a pillow should be placed under the stomach and hips to help keep the back straight.

REFERENCES

1. Bowerman, W. J., and Harris, W. D. *Jogging.* New York: Grosset and Dunlap, 1967.
2. Broer, M. R. *Efficiency of human movement.* 3d ed. Philadelphia: W. B. Saunders, 1973.
3. Bunn, J. W. *Scientific principles of coaching.* Englewood Cliffs, N.J.: Prentice-Hall, 1955.
4. Mathews, D. K., and Fox, E. L. *The physiological basis of physical education and athletics.* 2d ed. Philadelphia: W. B. Saunders, 1976.
5. Metheny, E. *Body dynamics.* New York: McGraw-Hill, 1952.
6. Scott, M. G. *Analysis of human motion.* 2d ed. New York: Appleton-Century-Crofts, 1963.
7. Wells, K. F. *Kinesiology.* Philadelphia: W. B. Saunders, 1971.
8. Wessel, J. *Movement fundamentals.* 2d ed. Englewood Cliffs, N.J.: Prentice-Hall, 1961.

CHAPTER ELEVEN
SUMMARY

In this book, the authors have attempted to provide the reader with information about human response to a regular exercise program (training), the benefits as well as the risks associated with engagement in such a program, and some of the biological and psychological consequences of failure to remain physically active throughout life. Exposure to this information should convince the reader to make a commitment to a lifetime exercise program.

This program should be based on sound scientific principles and should be developed to meet the needs of each individual. A summary of these principles and the procedures for development of an exercise program are provided below.

For persons under age 35 with no previous history of cardiovascular disease and without any of the CHD primary risk factors, no medical clearance is required prior to participation in a physical exercise program. All persons over age 35 are advised to receive medical clearance before they begin training.

Once the individual has determined that there are no contraindications to an exercise program, a personal fitness goal should be established and either a graded exercise test or a self-evaluation technique for circulorespiratory endurance should be administered. A physical exercise program can then be planned with consideration given to (1) the type of exercise to be conducted, (2) the frequency of training, and (3) the desired intensity and duration of each work period.

The type of exercise program is dictated by the particular components of physical fitness that the person wishes to develop or maintain—circulorespiratory endurance, muscular endurance and strength, flexibility, and weight management. Ideally, a regular exercise program would emphasize all these components. However, if one cannot devote enough time and effort to pursue an all-encompassing program, the components of circulorespiratory endurance, flexibility, and weight management should take precedence.

Circulorespiratory endurance is developed through aerobic activities, for example, running, walking, swimming, or bicycling for a relatively long distance or jumping rope for an extended period. The individual should select an aerobic activity or activities that he or she enjoys and one to which he or she can make a commitment to continue. Running is the best aerobic activity for development and maintenance of circulorespiratory endurance, although some people find it boring. In addition, individuals with joint problems (in the back, knees, and ankles) and foot disorders are unable to run for an extended period. Aside from the other activities just mentioned, singles play in tennis, racquetball, or handball are excellent alternatives to running if the participants have enough skill to produce continuous play or rallies. Unless both players have a moderate degree of skill, there usually is not enough movement in these sports to develop circulorespiratory endurance. Sports such as golf and bowling definitely do not require sufficient physical intensity to achieve that objective.

An exercise program designed to develop circulorespiratory endurance should be performed a minimum of 3 (nonconsecutive) days per week; however, a daily program is preferable. Many individuals exercise 5 to 7 days per week but prefer to modify the intensity or the duration or both on alternate days—they exercise with greater intensity and for a longer period every other day, or 3 or 4 days per week.

Determining the intensity at which one should exercise is difficult; however, if training effects are to occur, the principle of overload must be observed. Sedentary persons who initiate an exercise program should begin at a relatively low intensity and gradually increase the level of exertion. With great expectations of physical development, many persons undertake a program but they mistakenly begin their activity at an intensity that is too high for them. Their efforts result in soreness and discomfort, which hinder continuation of the program, and, upon recovery from the soreness, these persons have no desire to resume.

Monitoring the heart rate is the easiest method of determining the intensity at which one is working. Unless advised differently by a qualified physician, one should exercise at a minimum of 60% of one's maximum heart rate range. As the level of circulorespiratory endurance increases, this percentage can be increased. The heart rate can be used to indicate the intensity of all aerobic activities.

The duration of each exercise period is determined by the objectives of the program. The individual should devote 5 to 10 minutes to flexibility exercises and a minimum of 15 minutes to aerobic activity. As the level of circulorespiratory endurance improves, the duration of the exercise period can and perhaps should be increased.

It is well known that flexibility is specific to particular joints and to particular sports and that it decreases during the aging process; therefore, the individual should maintain a flexibility program for the entire body, with special emphasis on neck and shoulder flexibility, back extension, hip flexion, and posterior leg extension. Participants in a regular exercise program should be aware that many aerobic activities do not contribute to flexibility and, in fact, can actually decrease it; for example, jogging decreases the flexibility of the posterior upper and lower leg muscles. For all these reasons, static stretching daily, or at least 5 days per week, is recommended. In addition, sets of stretching for each specific flexibility should be performed several times throughout the day rather than all at once.

Weight management involves a combination of diet and exercise because caloric intake must be balanced by caloric expenditure (energy needs). It has been demonstrated that a combination of decreased caloric intake and increased physical activity is the most effective procedure for weight loss. The distance one walks, runs, bicycles, or swims, rather than the intensity of performance, is important for weight loss. The same number of calories is utilized whether one walks or runs for a specified distance. For effective development of circulorespiratory endurance and weight management, one should consider both the intensity and the duration of the exercise program.

Participation in a regular exercise program must be based on a personal decision. Excuses that are often given for not doing so—lack of time, of facilities, of motivation—should be reexamined in relation to the benefits of such a program. To enhance the quality of life, everyone should make regular, vigorous exercise a lifetime commitment.

APPENDIX A

COOPER'S TWELVE-MINUTE RUN

Cooper's Twelve-Minute Run is a test of circulorespiratory function. It should be performed **only** after the safety precautions (contraindications to exercise) described in Chapter 3 have been read.

The object of the test is to run, jog, or walk as far as possible during a 12-minute period. The distance is measured either in miles or in laps around the perimeter of a 94-foot by 50-foot rectangle. One lap equals 288 feet. It is calculated that an additional 12 feet are added where the runner turns the four corners so that one lap is actually at least 300 feet.

For a complete set of instructions for the test, see Laboratory 5.

Table A-1 converts laps to miles and assigns fitness categories based on the test. Table A-2 lists percentile scores for the test.

TABLE A-1
FITNESS CATEGORIES BASED ON COOPER'S
TWELVE-MINUTE RUN

Category	Laps*	Miles	$\dot{V}O_2$ (in ml/kg/min)†
Men			
Excellent	30.8 or more	1.75 or more	51.6 or greater
Good	26.4-30.7	1.50-1.74	42.6-51.5
Fair	22.0-26.3	1.25-1.49	33.8-42.5
Poor	21.9 or fewer	1.24 or fewer	33.7 or less
Women			
Excellent	29.0 or more	1.65 or more	. . . .
Good	23.8-28.9	1.35-1.64	. . . .
Fair	20.2-23.7	1.15-1.34	. . . .
Poor	20.1 or fewer	1.14 or fewer	. . . .

SOURCE: Kenneth H. Cooper, *The new aerobics* (New York: M. Evans, 1970).
*Assuming 17.6 laps per mile.
† No data available for women.

TABLE A-2
PERCENTILE SCORES FOR COOPER'S TWELVE-MINUTE RUN

	Men			Women	
Laps	Yards	%tile	Laps	Yards	%tile
35	3500	100.0	28	2800	100.0
34	3400	97.5	27	2700	97.0
33	3300	95.0	26	2600	94.0
32	3200	92.5	25	2500	91.0
31	3100	90.0	24	2400	88.0
30	3000	87.5	23	2300	85.0
29	2900	85.0	22	2200	82.0
28	2800	82.5	21	2100	79.0
27	2700	80.0	20	2000	76.0
26	2600	77.5	19	1900	73.0
25	2500	75.0	18	1800	70.0
24	2400	72.5	17	1700	67.0
23	2300	70.0	16	1600	64.0
22	2200	67.5	15	1500	61.0
21	2100	65.0			
20	2000	62.5			
19	1900	60.0			

NOTE: These scores are developed for indoor administration of the test with laps around a standard basketball court (94 ft x 50 ft).

APPENDIX B

SAMPLE EXERCISE PRESCRIPTION

Name: _Scott Burgess_ Age: _19_ Exercise preference: _Jogging_

Resting HR: _75_ Max HR: _195_ Training HR: 60% _147_; 70% _159_;

80% _171_

CR evaluation by _12-min run_ Results: _Fair (1.3 miles)_

Comments: _Negligible regular physical activity during previous 3_
years.

Fitness goal: _Run 3 miles continuously at 8.5 min/mile pace_
without undue stress.

EXERCISE RECOMMENDATIONS

General: _Precede all exercise sessions with warm-up of light calis-_
thenics and flexibility exercises. End all workouts with 10
to 15 min of cool-down activities before entering a
warmer environment. Use caution when exercising in
adverse environmental conditions (e.g., high heat and
humidity).

Specific:

Exercise style & type: _Continuous activity—walk/jog— eventu-_
ally full jog at 8.5 min/mile pace.

Frequency: _Initially triweekly, symmetrically spaced. After 3 to_
5 weeks, increase to 4 to 5 workouts/week if
desired.

Intensity: _60% to 75% of max HR range._

Duration: _20 min/workout initially (excluding warm-up and_
cool-down). After 8 to 10 weeks increase to 30 to 40
min if desired.

GLOSSARY

Adenosine Diphosphate. A compound (ester) composed of one molecule each of adenine and D-ribose and two molecules of phosphoric acid. It is formed as a result of the breakdown of adenosine triphosphate and is used in the resynthesis of adenosine triphosphate.

Adenosine triphosphate. A compound (ester) composed of one molecule each of adenine and D-ribose and three molecules of phosphoric acid. Its breakdown by hydrolysis is accompanied by the release of energy for muscular and other types of cellular activity.

Adrenal glands. Endocrine glands, one located immediately above each kidney. They produce epinephrine and norepinephrine and many steroidal hormones involved in electrolyte and fluid balance.

Aerobic power (aerobic capacity). The capacity of one's heart, lungs, and vascular system to deliver oxygen to working muscles.

Asymptomatic. Presenting none of the symptoms usually connected with the identification of particular diseases.

Baroreceptors. Nerve endings in various arteries that respond to pressure (e.g., blood pressure, stretching, touching).

Beriberi. A disease caused by deficiency of thiamine (vitamin B_1). It is characterized by cardiovascular abnormalities, edema, and cerebral manifestations and other nerve damage.

Body image. The feelings and attitudes an individual has towards his or her body.

Catecholamines. One of a group of similar compounds that mimic responses to activity of the sympathetic nervous system. Examples are epinephrine and norepinephrine.

Distributed practice. A system of practice schedules that are separated by either rest or some activity that is different from the one being practiced.

Dynamic contraction. Isotonic contraction: a type of muscle contraction in which shortening of the muscle fibers occurs. Movement is involved.

Eccentric contraction. A type of muscle contraction in which there is a gradual lengthening of the muscle fibers from a shortened position against resistance.

Extracellular fluid. Fluid that is found outside of the cells of the body.

Fibrinolysis. The activity of the fibrinolysin system, which removes small clots from tiny vessels throughout the body.

Glucose. A simple sugar belonging to the monosaccharide group, which is oxidized in the body to liberate heat and energy.

Glycogen. Animal starch, which is stored in the animal body for future conversion into sugar (glucose) and for subsequent use as a source of energy.

Hemodynamic. Related to circulation or to the cardiovascular system.

Histological. Pertaining to microscopic structure.

Homeostatic balance. The presence of physiological equilibrium in which body functions and conditions are within an acceptable and safe range.

Hyperextension. Extreme extension or overextension of a joint of the body.

Hypokinetic disease. Malady due to lack of movement.

Interventricular septum. Tissue that separates the left side of the heart from the right side.

Intracellular fluid. Fluid that is found within the cell wall.

Isokinetic contraction. A type of muscular contraction in which the speed of the contraction and the resistance encountered are unchanged during the entire range of motion.

Isometric contraction. Static contraction: a type of muscle contraction in which no shortening of the muscle fibers occurs, which thus produces no movement.

Isotonic contraction. See **Dynamic contraction.**

IU. International unit, a quantity of a substance (e.g., a vitamin) that produces a particular biological effect agreed upon as an international standard.

Lactacid. The portion of an oxygen debt in which lactic acid is accumulated. This portion is repaid very slowly.

Lactic acid. A by-product of anaerobic metabolism which results from the incomplete oxidation of glucose during muscular work. It is capable of terminating muscular contraction if its concentration is high enough.

Lesion. Any pathological or traumatic discontinuity of tissue or loss of function of a part.

Lipid. Any one of a group of organic substances that are insoluble in water but soluble in alcohol, ether, chloroform, and other fat solvents. It has a greasy feel.

Massed practice. A system of practice schedules that have little or no rest or alternate activity between the beginning and the end of the activity being practiced.

MET. The metabolic equivalent of resting oxygen uptake expressed in terms of milliliters per kilogram of body weight per minute.

Metabolism. The sum of all the physical and chemical processes by which living organized substance is produced and maintained; also, the transformation by which energy is made available for the uses of an organism.

Motor Nerves. Fibers of tissue that conduct impulses from the brain to the muscle tissue. The impulse must be transmitted if movement is to take place.

Murmur (heart). One of various sounds produced by the heart during specific events of the cardiac cycle, usually the result of a leaky or narrowed valve. It may or may not be pathologic.

Neuritis. Inflammation of a nerve or nerves, which is marked by pain, sensory disturbances, and impaired reflexes.

Neuromuscular efficiency. Control of the muscles by the motor-nerve stimuli in the least wasteful manner.

Oxygen consumption. The amount of oxygen processed by the body. It is usually expressed in liters per minute but sometimes expressed in milliliters per kilogram of body weight per minute, to allow interpersonal comparisons to be made. Also called **oxygen intake** and **oxygen uptake.**

Oxygen extraction. The amount of oxygen extracted from 100 ml of blood.

Palpation. The act of feeling with the hand by light finger pressure.

Peripheral circulation. Blood flow through small vessels surrounded by muscles.

Pernicious anemia. A progressive decrease in the number and increase in the size of red blood cells, which results in weakness and gastrointestinal and nervous disturbances.

Relaxation. The relief or reduction of tension in the body. It reduces muscle tonus.

Repetition max (RM). The maximum number of times that one can repeat an exercise with a specified amount of weight.

Self-concept. An individual's perception of the kind of person he or she is.

Self-estimate. An individual's success or failure as defined by himself or herself.

Self-image. An individual's view of himself or herself at a particular time and place.

Static contraction. See **Isometric contraction.**

Stress. Any situation in which the body's homeostatic balance is disturbed.

Stressor. Any psychological or physical condition that disturbs the homeostatic balance of the body; anything that causes stress.

Stretch reflex. The reflex contraction of a muscle in response to being suddenly stretched beyond its normal length. This reflex action serves to prevent injury due to overstretching.

Sympathetic nervous system. A division of the autonomic, or involuntary, nervous system, which is responsible for promoting the body's reactions to a stressor.

Symptomatic. Presenting symptoms of a known condition, usually pathologic.

Tension. Increased muscle tonus, in which the muscles are contracted more than is necessary to maintain posture.

Viscera. Internal organs.

Work-relief ratio. The proportion between time spent working and time spent recovering. A work-relief ratio of 1:2 means that the recovery period is twice as long as the work period.

INDEX

Laboratory 1

KNOWLEDGE AND ATTITUDE ABOUT THE PURPOSE AND VALUE OF PHYSICAL ACTIVITY

Name _____   Instructor _____

Class and section _____   Date _____

Purpose

The purpose of this laboratory session is to evaluate your knowledge and attitude about the purpose and value of physical activity.

Equipment Needed

None

Procedure

Read each of the 45 items listed below and check yes or no the answer that best indicates your knowledge or attitude.

Yes　**No**

_____　_____　1. Do you avoid the use of labor-saving devices whenever possible (e.g., riding lawn mowers and riding golf carts)?

_____　_____　2. Do you regularly perform work that requires vigorous physical exertion?

_____　_____　3. Do you regularly (at least three times per week) participate in physically active lifetime sports (e.g., tennis, racquetball, handball, or badminton)?

_____　_____　4. Do you regularly (at least three times per week) participate in aerobic activities that involve a minimum of 20 minutes of continuous movement (e.g., jogging, jumping rope, bicycling, or swimming)?

Yes   No

_____   _____   5. Do you believe that you can jog 2 miles and continue your daily activities without experiencing fatigue in the evening?

_____   _____   6. Do you know the guidelines and precautions that should be followed when you first begin an exercise program?

_____   _____   7. Can you plan an exercise program for a 40-year-old sedentary individual?

_____   _____   8. Are you able to describe the benefits of a regular exercise program?

_____   _____   9. Are you able to estimate the energy expenditure of various physical activities?

_____   _____   10. Do you know the differences among circuit, interval, and aerobic training?

_____   _____   11. Are you able to develop an individualized training program for strength improvement?

_____   _____   12. Are you able to identify the primary and secondary risk factors associated with the development of coronary heart disease?

_____   _____   13. Are you able to identify safe ranges for blood pressure, serum cholesterol, and serum triglycerides?

_____   _____   14. Are you able to describe the role of exercise in the prevention of, and the rehabilitation after, coronary heart disease?

_____   _____   15. Are you able to select and self-administer a suitable test for classification of the functional capacity of the circulorespiratory system?

_____   _____   16. Are you able to determine your target heart rate for training?

Yes   **No**

_____   _____   17.   Are you able to state the physiological adaptations to endurance training and to strength training?

_____   _____   18.   Are you able to develop an individualized training program for the improvement of circulorespiratory endurance?

_____   _____   19.   Are you aware of the problems and disorders associated with the lack of flexibility?

_____   _____   20.   Are you able to determine your flexibility in the neck, shoulder, chest, trunk, lower back, hips, and hamstring muscles?

_____   _____   21.   Are you able to design an individualized program to develop flexibility?

_____   _____   22.   Do you know the major reasons why individuals are overweight?

_____   _____   23.   Do you know the effects of being overweight?

_____   _____   24.   Do you know the difference between saturated and unsaturated fat?

_____   _____   25.   Are you able to describe an adequate diet in relation to carbohydrate, protein, and fat percentages?

_____   _____   26.   Are you able to describe a weight reduction plan in relation to caloric intake and exercise?

_____   _____   27.   Do you know the characteristics of a tense individual?

_____   _____   28.   Can you identify any stress-related diseases and disorders?

_____   _____   29.   Can you describe the role of exercise in helping to prevent stress-related disorders?

_____   _____   30.   Are you able to release tension through a relaxation technique?

Yes	No		
____	____	31.	Are you able to state the maximum normal values for heart rate and systolic blood pressure?
____	____	32.	Are you able to describe the changes in respiratory function that result from long-term endurance training?
____	____	33.	Are you able to describe good posture and movement mechanics for standing, running for distance, lifting, and sitting?
____	____	34.	Do you avoid the use of alcohol and tranquilizers after a stressful experience or a bad day?
____	____	35.	Do you believe you have good eating habits?
____	____	36.	Are you able to relax immediately when you go to bed at night?
____	____	37.	Do you enjoy social interaction through participation in sports?
____	____	38.	Do you have a socially acceptable way of releasing aggressive drives and hostile feelings?
____	____	39.	Is your typical day free from an unusual number of stressful experiences?
____	____	40.	Have you avoided any weight gain during the past year?
____	____	41.	Do you believe you have good posture when walking and sitting?
____	____	42.	Do you know the relationship of percentage of body fat and acceptable body weight?
____	____	43.	Do you like yourself?
____	____	44.	Do you enjoy mental and physical challenge?
____	____	45.	Are you physically fit?

Results

In today's society most people need to participate in a regular physical activity program; however, many fail to do so due to their lack of knowledge about the value of physical fitness and their attitude toward physical activity. Observe how many questions you answered no. These answers may indicate a lack of knowledge about and a negative attitude toward physical activity.

Do you believe that an increased knowledge about the value of physical fitness and participation in a regular physical activity program can change a negative attitude toward physical activity?

———————————

Laboratory 2

FLEXIBILITY EVALUATION

Name _____   Instructor _____

Class and section _____   Date _____

PURPOSE

The purpose of this laboratory session is to evaluate your flexibility in the neck, shoulders and shoulder girdle, chest muscles, trunk extension, trunk and hips, lower back and hips, and hamstring muscles.

Equipment Needed

1. Bench
2. Ruler or yardstick

Procedures

1. Take the flexibility tests described on pp. 70-73.
2. Report the first three tests (shoulder lift, trunk extension, and sit and reach) in inches. Report the remaining four tests as passed (P) or failed (F).
3. Use Table 5-1 (p. 72) to determine your flexibility classification for the first three tests.

Test	Score	Classification
Shoulder Lift (Fig. 5-1, p. 71)	_____	_____
Trunk Extension (Fig. 5-2, p. 71)	_____	_____
Sit and Reach (Fig. 5-3, p. 72)	_____	_____
Neck Flexibility (Fig. 5-4, p. 73)	_____	_____
Hips and Lower Back (Fig. 5-5, p. 73)	_____	_____
Hamstring Muscles (Fig. 5-6, p. 73)	_____	_____
Chest Muscles (Fig. 5-7, p. 73)	_____	_____

Results

Flexibility is not a general factor, but is specific to given joints and sports or physical activities. Active individuals tend to be more flexible than inactive individuals. Do you need to develop additional flexibility? _____

Laboratory 3

FLEXIBILITY EXERCISES

Name _____   Instructor _____

Class and section _____   Date _____

Purpose

The purposes of this laboratory session are:
1. To provide the opportunity to practice the flexibility exercises described on pp. 74-91.
2. To guide you in the formation of a flexibility program that can be conducted throughout your lifetime.

Equipment Needed

Towels

Procedures

Perform each of the flexibility exercises described on pp. 74-91. Follow all the instructions concerning duration and mechanics.

Results

1. Did you experience difficulty with any of the exercises? _____

2. Do you believe you should perform certain flexibility exercises daily? _____

3. What do you think will happen to your flexibility as you grow older? _____

It is impossible to state how much flexibility is desirable; however, everyone should strive to prevent loss of flexibility because the lack of it can create disorders or functional problems.

Laboratory 4

ESTIMATION OF
HEART ATTACK RISK

Name _____   Instructor _____

Class and section _____   Date _____

Purpose

The purpose of this laboratory session is to provide you with an estimate of your chances of suffering a heart attack now and in the future. You will make this estimate by playing the game RISKO.

Equipment Needed

1. Sphygmomanometer
2. Stethoscope
3. RISKO Game Card and Score Sheet

Procedure

1. Play the game as the directions indicate for your present age. (See pp. 208-210.)
2. Play the game a second time with data you estimate to be descriptive of your mother (for women) or your father (for men).

Results

1. What is your RISKO score? _____

2. What is your RISKO classification? _____

3. What is your parents' score? _____

4. What is your parents' classification? _____

5. List the factors that you might be able to change to decrease your chances of suffering a heart attack.

RISKO

The purpose of this game is to give you an estimate of your chances of suffering heart attack.

The game is played by marking squares which—from left to right—represent an increase in your risk factors. These are medical conditions and habits associated with an increased danger of heart attack. *Not all risk factors are measurable enough to be included in this game.*

Rules:

Study each risk factor and its row. Find the box applicable to you and circle the large number in it. For example, if you are 37, circle the number in the box labeled 31-40.

After checking out all the rows, add the circled numbers. This total—your score—is an estimate of your risk.

If you score:

6-11 — Risk well below average
12-17 — Risk below average
18-24 — Risk generally average
25-31 — Risk moderate
32-40 — Risk at a dangerous level
41-62 — Danger urgent. See your doctor now.

Heredity:

Count parents, grandparents, brothers, and sisters who have had heart attack and/or stroke.

Tobacco smoking:

If you inhale deeply and smoke a cigarette way down, add one to your classification. Do not subtract because you think you do not inhale or smoke only a half inch on a cigarette.

Exercise

Lower your score one point if you exercise regularly and frequently.

Reproduced with permission of the Michigan Heart Association.

Cholesterol or saturated fat intake level:

A cholesterol blood test is best. If you can't get one from your doctor, then estimate honestly the percentage of solid fats you eat. These are usually of animal origin—lard, cream, butter, and beef and lamb fat. If you eat much of this, your cholesterol level probably will be high. The U.S. average, 40%, is too high for good health.

Blood pressure:

If you have no recent reading but have passed an insurance or industrial examination, chances are you are 140 or less.

Sex:

This line takes into account the fact that men have from 6 to 10 times more heart attacks than women of childbearing age.

RISKO SCORE

Name _____ Sex _____ Date _____

Place the correct score for each factor on the appropriate line.

	Yourself	Dad or Mom
Age		
Heredity		
Weight		
Tobacco smoking		
Exercise		
Cholesterol or fat percentage in diet		
Blood pressure		
Sex		
Total		
Classification		

Age	**1** 10 to 20	**2** 21 to 30	**3** 31 to 40	**4** 41 to 50	**6** 51 to 60	**8** 61 to 70 and over
Heredity	**1** No known history of heart disease	**2** 1 relative with cardiovascular disease Over 60	**3** 2 relatives with cardiovascular disease Over 60	**4** 1 relative with cardiovascular disease Under 60	**6** 2 relatives with cardiovascular disease Under 60	**7** 3 relatives with cardiovascular disease Under 60
Weight	**0** More than 5 lb below standard weight	**1** −5 to +5 lb standard weight	**2** 6–20 lb over-weight	**3** 21–35 lb over-weight	**5** 36–50 lb over-weight	**7** 51–65 lb over-weight
Tobacco smoking	**0** Non-user	**1** Cigar and/or pipe	**2** 10 cigarettes or less a day	**4** 20 cigarettes a day	**6** 30 cigarettes a day	**10** 40 cigarettes a day or more
Exercise	**1** Intensive occupational & recreational exertion	**2** Moderate occupational & recreational exertion	**3** Sedentary work & intense recreational exertion	**5** Sedentary occupational and moderate exertion	**6** Sedentary work & light recreational exertion	**8** Complete lack of all exercise
Cholesterol or fat % in diet	**1** Cholesterol below 180 mg%. Diet contains no animal or solid fats	**2** Cholesterol 181–205 mg%. Diet contains 10% animal or solid fats	**3** Cholesterol 206–230 mg%. Diet contains 20% animal or solid fats	**4** Cholesterol 231–255 mg%. Diet contains 30% animal or solid fats	**5** Cholesterol 256–280 mg%. Diet contains 40% animal or solid fats	**7** Cholesterol 281–300 mg%. Diet contains 50% animal or solid fats
Blood pressure	**1** 100 upper reading	**2** 120 upper reading	**3** 140 upper reading	**4** 160 upper reading	**6** 180 upper reading	**8** 200 or over upper reading
Sex	**1** Female under 40	**2** Female 40-50	**3** Female over 50	**5** Male	**6** Stocky male	**7** Bald stocky male

Laboratory 5

EVALUATION OF CIRCULORESPIRATORY FITNESS (COOPER'S TWELVE-MINUTE RUN)

Name _____   Instructor _____

Class and section _____   Date _____

Purpose

The purpose of this laboratory session is to evaluate your present level of circulorespiratory fitness by means of Cooper's Twelve-Minute Run. This test is based on research that demonstrates that the distance one can cover in 12 minutes correlates very highly with the ability of one's body to use large amounts of oxygen.

Equipment Needed

1. Timing device that will run for 12 minutes consecutively
2. Method for measuring the distance covered
   This can be counted in miles or in laps around a rectangle 94 feet by 50 feet. One lap equals 288 feet. It is calculated that an additional 12 feet are added when a runner rounds off the four corners so that one lap is actually at least 300 feet.

Procedure

1. The objective of the participant is to cover as much distance as possible in the allowed 12-minute period.
2. Start the timer, then run, jog, or walk for 12 consecutive minutes.
3. Determine the distance covered in miles.
4. Refer to Table A-1 (see p. 185) to find your fitness level.
5. Alternative procedure: Construct a rectangle 94 feet by 50 feet. Run along the outside perimeter of this figure and count laps. Laps are converted to miles in Table A-1. Proceed as in step 4.

Results

1. What distance did you cover? _____

2. On the basis of this test, what is your fitness category? _____

3. Are you pleased, satisfied, or dissatisfied with the results? _____

4. Do you believe that more experience in how to establish a pace would help improve your score? _____

5. Do you believe that this test accurately reflects your present level of circulorespiratory fitness? _____

Scores for additional 12-minute runs:

Date	Laps (Distance)	Score
_____	_____	_____
_____	_____	_____
_____	_____	_____
_____	_____	_____
_____	_____	_____

Laboratory 6

EVALUATION OF CIRCULORESPIRATORY FITNESS (HARVARD STEP TEST)

Name _____   Instructor _____

Class and section _____   Date _____

Purpose

The purpose of this laboratory session is to evaluate your circulorespiratory fitness by means of the Harvard Step Test. This test is based on the fact that the speed at which you recover from hard exercise is a reliable indicator of your level of circulorespiratory fitness.

Equipment Needed

1. One sturdy 20-inch bench; one sturdy 18-inch bench
   If gymnasium bleachers are to be used, 2-inch by 6-inch boards bolted into place on top of the seat increase the step height sufficiently to permit substitution for the 20-inch bench.
2. Metronome
3. Timer with a second hand that will run for 8.5 minutes consecutively

Procedure

The male subject steps up and down on the 20-inch bench 30 times per minute for 5 minutes. The female steps up and down on the 18-inch bench 30 times per minute for 4 minutes.

At the end of the test, the subject sits immediately. The pulse is counted and recorded during 30-second intervals after 1 minute, 2 minutes, and 3 minutes of recovery. Use the following score sheet to calculate your score for the test.

	Recovery Period	Pulse Count
1 to 1.5 min		_____
2 to 2.5 min		_____
3 to 3.5 min		_____
Sum of 3 pulse counts		_____

Long Form

$$\text{Index} = \frac{(\text{duration of exercise in seconds}) \times 100}{2 \times (\text{sum of pulse counts during recovery})}$$

$$= \frac{(\underline{\hspace{1cm}}) \times 100}{2 \times (\underline{\hspace{1cm}})}$$

$$= \underline{\hspace{3cm}}$$

$$\text{Index} = \underline{\hspace{3cm}}$$

Short Form

$$\text{Index} = \frac{(\text{duration of exercise in seconds}) \times 100}{5.5 \times (\text{pulse count, 1 to 1.5 min})}$$

$$= \frac{(\underline{\hspace{1cm}}) \times 100}{5.5 \times (\underline{\hspace{1cm}})}$$

$$= \underline{\hspace{3cm}}$$

$$\text{Index} = \underline{\hspace{3cm}}$$

Classification

Below 55	Poor
55–64	Low average
65–79	Average
80–89	Good
90 and above	Excellent

Results

1. What is your classification? _____

2. How do the results of this test compare with your performance on the 12-minute run? _____

3. Which test do you perceive to be physically more demanding?
   _____

4. Are you pleased or displeased with your score? _____

Laboratory 7

CAROTID PULSE MONITORING AND TARGET HEART RATE DURING TRAINING

Name _____ Instructor _____

Class and section _____ Date _____

Purpose

The purposes of this laboratory session are to practice palpation of the carotid pulse, to determine how high you must elevate your heart rate to achieve a training stimulus, and to get a feel for a training pace that elicits your target heart rate.

Equipment

Stopwatch or wristwatch with a second hand

Procedure

1. Use the first two fingers on your preferred hand to find your carotid artery. (See Figure 3-2.)
2. Press lightly until you can feel your carotid pulse.
3. Count your pulse for 10 seconds, then multiply by 6 to get your heart rate for 1 minute.
4. Try this several times during a 10-minute rest period while you are either seated or reclining.
5. Assume that the lowest value obtained is your resting heart rate and calculate your exercise target heart rate as follows:

Example

a. Predicted maximum heart rate* = _____   _____ 200

b. Resting heart rate = - _____   - 70

* Subtract your age from 220 for predicted maximum HR if actual value is not known.

215

			Example
c.	Maximum heart rate range	= _____	130
d.	Percentage of MHR range for training (60%, 70%, 80%)	= × _____	× 0.60
e.	Multiply step *c* times the desired value from step *d*	= _____	78
f.	Resting heart rate	= + _____	+ 70
g.	Target heart rate for training	= _____	148
h.	Calculate your training range 60% to 75% (LSD)	= _____	
i.	Calculate your training range 80% to 85% (interval)	= _____	

6. Now jog slowly for 3 minutes. Stop and immediately count your carotid pulse for 10 seconds.
7. If the intensity of the exercise was too light, the rate will be lower than the desired rate. If this is the case, jog a little faster for 3 more minutes and take your pulse rate again. Continue until you have found the pace at which you must work.

Results

Once you develop a feel for your own pace, you should be able to maintain the desired rate comfortably for 10 to 15 minutes. After a few training sessions, you will need to reexamine your resting heart rate to see if a new target rate is to be determined. In each training session, it is desirable to monitor your heart rate both during and immediately after the exercise to insure an adequate level of intensity for training.

Laboratory 8

INTERVAL TRAINING

Name _____   Instructor _____

Class and section _____   Date _____

Purpose

The purpose of this laboratory session is to demonstrate the use of interval (intermittent) training, as might be used indoors or outdoors in a relatively small area.

Equipment Needed

1. Timing device with a second hand, such as a wall clock, lab timer, stopwatch, or wristwatch
2. Marked area approximately 94 feet by 50 feet (the size of an official basketball court)

Procedure

Progress through an interval-style workout as outlined below. The work consists of a series of activities that are interspaced with recovery periods. The work will become progressively harder, will reach a peak, and then will taper off.

1. Begin with 3 to 5 minutes of stretching and flexibility exercises as described on pp. 74-91.
2. Walk 2 laps (L) around the perimeter of the basketball court (or a rectangle 94 feet by 50 feet) at a vigorous pace.
3. Walk 1L at a vigorous pace while you make swimming movements with your arms.
4. Racing-walk 0.5L, then walk regularly the remainder of the lap.
5. Walk 1L very slowly.
6. Jog 1L very slowly.
7. Walk 1L to recover.
8. Jog 1L at a moderate pace (25 to 30 seconds per lap).
9. Walk 1L to recover.
10. Jog 1L at a moderate pace.
11. Walk 1L to recover.
12. Jog 2L at a moderate pace. Walk 1L to recover.

13. Jog 3L. Walk 1L to recover.
    Note: Check heart rate during the first 10 seconds after jogging 3L and remember the value. (HR should be in 60% to 70% range.)

14. At center court, execute the following high-intensity exercises consecutively. No rest intervals. Exercises are to be executed as fast as possible!
    a. Running, in place, knees waist-high for 15 seconds
    b. 10 push-ups
    c. Repeat step a
    d. Supine flutter kicking for 15 seconds
    e. Repeat step a
    f. Prone flutter kicking for 15 seconds
    g. Repeat step a
    h. 10 sit-ups
    i. Repeat step a
    j. 10 squat jumps
    k. Repeat step a
    l. Check heart rate immediately (HR should be in 80% to 85% range.)

15. Walk 1L to recover.
16. Jog 3L at a moderate pace. Walk 1L to recover.
17. Jog 2L at a moderate pace. Walk 1L to recover.
18. Jog 1L. Walk 3L to recover.
19. Cool down for 5 to 10 minutes before a shower.

Results

This program produces varying degrees of stress depending on (1) how vigorously the steps are executed and (2) the physical condition of the participant. If your heart rate was not within the 60% to 70% range at the end of step 13, you should (1) increase the pace (e.g., to 20 seconds per lap) and (2) increase the number of consecutive laps (e.g., to 4L or 5L) before you proceed to the high-intensity exercises. After the high-intensity exercises (step 14) are completed, your heart rate should be at least as high as your target heart rate (85%) as calculated by Karvonen's method. (See p. 37.) In the early stages of training, most people prefer to intersperse work with frequent rest periods. As your body adapts to the repeated stress over a period of days or weeks, you will need to increase the stimulus by (1) increasing the pace, (2) progressively increasing the number of consecutive laps, or (3) removing the recovery laps to make the program more continuous than intermittent.

Laboratory 9

CIRCUIT TRAINING FOR STRENGTH

Name _____   Instructor _____

Class and section _____   Date _____

Purpose

The purpose of this laboratory session is to demonstrate a modification of the circuit-training approach as applied to strength training.

Equipment Needed

A Universal Gym or some similar weight-training apparatus

Procedure

1. Determine the maximum amount of weight that can be handled through five repetitions (5 RM) of each of the following exercises:
   a. Leg curls
   b. Weighted chins
   c. Leg press
   d. Bench press
   e. Weighted sit-ups
   f. Military press
2. Begin with step 1a. Complete the 5 RM.
3. Proceed to step 1b. Repeat the 5 RM.
4. Continue the pattern until all steps (a through f) have been completed three times (three sets). Note: In the second and third sets, initially you might not be able to complete 5 RM owing to fatigue. As you increase in strength, you will find that you can do much beyond the initial 5 RM, particularly in the first set. To keep the work uniformly distributed over the three sets, you must adhere to the following regulations.
   a. Do not exceed eight repetitions in the first or second sets no matter how strong you feel.

b. If you execute eight repetitions in the first and second sets and you can exceed eight repetitions in the third set of a particular exercise, you must establish a new 5 RM for that lift. To find the new 5 RM, simply add weight until five repetitions are once again the maximum you can lift without a pause for rest.

c. Remember to stagger the lifts so that the same muscle groups are not used in successive exercises.

Results

This type of weight training is very strenuous and should be engaged in only triweekly on nonconsecutive days. As the resistance increases, you may need some slight assistance to overcome the inertia of a weight at rest.

Laboratory 10

BODY FRAME AND DESIRABLE BODY WEIGHT

Name _____   Instructor _____

Class and section _____   Date _____

Purpose

The purpose of this laboratory session is to estimate your body-frame size and desirable body weight.

Equipment Needed

1. Measurement tape
2. Scales

Procedures

1. Estimate your body-frame size (small, medium, or large) with the technique described on p. 118.
2. Estimate your desirable body weight with Table 6-1.
3. Use the OW index described on p. 118 to estimate whether you are overweight. Values of 100 or less are considered to indicate a good weight, and values greater than 110 are considered to indicate overweight.

Ankle girth measurement _____

Body frame _____

Weight _____

Height _____

OW index _____

Results

Desirable body weight is best estimated through measurement of the percentage of body fat. Is your weight acceptable to you as compared with the standards given above? _____

Laboratory 11

ESTIMATION OF
BODY-FAT PERCENTAGE

Name _____   Instructor _____

Class and section _____   Date _____

Purpose

The purpose of this laboratory session is to estimate your percentage of body fat.

Equipment Needed

Skinfold calipers

Procedure

1. Have your skinfold thicknesses measured as described on pp. 119-122.
2. Use the appropriate formula on pp. 224-225 or Tables 1 or 2 provided in this exercise to estimate your percentage of body fat. _____ = % fat.

Results

1. Use 15% for males and 20% for females as the upper normal limit of body fat. Are you above normal, below normal, or about right in percentage of body fat? _____
2. To determine your fat weight (FW), use the following formula:

$$FW = body\ weight\ \times\ \%\ fat$$

$$= \underline{\hspace{2cm}} \times \underline{\hspace{1cm}}$$

$$FW = \underline{\hspace{2cm}} lb$$

3. To determine your lean body weight (LBW), use the following formula:

$$LBW = body\ weight\ -\ FW$$

$$= \underline{\hspace{2cm}} lb\ -\ \underline{\hspace{1.5cm}} lb$$

$$LBW = \underline{\hspace{2.5cm}} lb$$

4. If you wish to reduce your fat weight, you can determine your target body weight (TBW) by using the following formula:

$$TBW = \frac{LBW}{1.00\ -\ desired\ \%\ fat}$$

$$= \underline{\hspace{3cm}}$$

$$TBW =$$

SAMPLE CALCULATION
OF PERCENTAGE OF BODY FAT

Step 1. Calculation of Body Density

For females,[*]

Body density = 1.0764−(0.00081 × skinfold thickness at iliac crest)
                      −(0.00088 × skinfold thickness at triceps)

Skinfold Site	Sample Thickness[†]	Actual Thickness[†]
Iliac crest	13 mm	_____ mm
Triceps	10 mm	_____ mm

Body density = 1.0764 − (0.00081 × 13) − (0.00088 × 10)
                      = 1.057

For males,[‡]

Body density = 1.1043 −(0.001327 × skinfold thickness at thigh)
                      −(0.001310 × skinfold thickness at scapula)

---

[*]A. W. Sloan, J. J. Burt, and C. S. Blyth, Estimation of body fat in young women, *Journal of Applied Physiology* 17:967–970, 1962.
[†]Average of two measurements.
[‡]A. W. Sloan, Estimation of body fat in young men, *Journal of Applied Physiology* 23:311–315, 1967.

Skinfold Site	**Sample Thickness†**	**Actual Thickness†**
Scapula	11 mm	_____ mm
Thigh	11 mm	_____ mm

Body density = $1.1043 - (0.001327 \times 11) - (0.001310 \times 11)$
= 1.0753

Step 2. Calculation of Percentage of Body Fat**

$$\text{Percentage of body fat} = \left(\frac{4.570}{\text{body density}} - 4.142 \right) \times 100$$

For the sample female,

$$\text{Percentage of body fat} = \frac{4.570}{1.057} - 4.142 = 0.182 = 18.2\%$$

For the sample male,

$$\text{Percentage of body fat} = \frac{4.570}{1.0753} - 4.142 = 0.108 = 10.8\%$$

†Average of two measurements.
**J. Brozek, F. Grande, J. T. Anderson, and A. Keys, Densitometric analysis of body composition: Revision of some quantitative assumptions, *Annals of the New York Academy of Science* 110:113–140, 1963.

**TABLE 1—MALES: CONVERSION
SKINFOLD MEASUREMENTS**

	Thigh skinfold																	
Skinfold thickness at scapula (in mm)	6	6.5	7	7.5	8	8.5	9	9.5	10	10.5	11	11.5	12	12.5	13	13.5	14	14.5
4	5	5	5	5	6	6	6	6	7	7	7	7	8	8	8	8	9	9
4.5	5	5	5	6	6	6	6	7	7	7	7	8	8	8	8	8	9	9
5	5	5	6	6	6	6	7	7	7	7	8	8	8	8	9	9	9	10
5.5	5	6	6	6	6	7	7	7	7	8	8	8	8	9	9	9	10	10
6	6	6	6	6	7	7	7	7	8	8	8	8	9	9	9	10	10	10
6.5	6	6	6	7	7	7	7	8	8	8	8	9	9	9	10	10	10	10
7	6	6	7	7	7	7	8	8	8	8	9	9	9	10	10	10	10	11
7.5	6	7	7	7	7	8	8	8	8	9	9	9	10	10	10	10	11	11
8	7	7	7	7	8	8	8	8	9	9	9	10	10	10	10	11	11	11
8.5	7	7	7	8	8	8	8	9	9	9	10	10	10	10	11	11	11	11
9	7	7	8	8	8	8	9	9	9	10	10	10	10	11	11	11	11	12
9.5	7	8	8	8	8	9	9	9	10	10	10	10	11	11	11	11	12	12
10	8	8	8	8	9	9	9	9	10	10	10	11	11	11	11	12	12	12
10.5	8	8	8	9	9	9	9	10	10	10	11	11	11	11	12	12	12	12
11	8	8	9	9	9	9	10	10	10	11	11	11	11	12	12	12	12	13
11.5	8	9	9	9	9	10	10	10	11	11	11	11	12	12	12	12	13	13
12	9	9	9	9	10	10	10	11	11	11	11	12	12	12	12	13	13	13
12.5	9	9	9	10	10	10	11	11	11	11	12	12	12	12	13	13	13	13
13	9	9	10	10	10	11	11	11	11	12	12	12	12	13	13	13	13	14
13.5	9	10	10	10	11	11	11	11	12	12	12	12	13	13	13	13	14	14
14	10	10	10	11	11	11	11	12	12	12	12	13	13	13	13	14	14	14
14.5	10	10	11	11	11	11	12	12	12	12	13	13	13	13	14	14	14	14
15	10	11	11	11	11	12	12	12	12	13	13	13	13	14	14	14	14	15
15.5	11	11	11	11	12	12	12	12	13	13	13	13	14	14	14	14	15	15
16	11	11	11	12	12	12	12	13	13	13	13	14	14	14	14	15	15	15
16.5	11	11	12	12	12	12	13	13	13	13	14	14	14	14	15	15	15	16
17	11	12	12	12	12	13	13	13	13	14	14	14	14	15	15	15	16	16
17.5	12	12	12	12	13	13	13	14	14	14	14	15	15	15	16	16	16	16
18	12	12	12	13	13	13	13	14	14	14	14	15	15	15	16	16	16	16
18.5	12	12	13	13	13	13	14	14	14	14	15	15	15	16	16	16	16	17
19	12	13	13	13	13	14	14	14	14	15	15	15	16	16	16	16	17	17
19.5	13	13	13	13	14	14	14	14	15	15	15	16	16	16	16	17	17	17
20	13	13	13	14	14	14	14	15	15	15	16	16	16	16	17	17	17	17
20.5	13	13	14	14	14	14	15	15	15	16	16	16	16	17	17	17	17	18
21	13	14	14	14	14	15	15	15	16	16	16	16	17	17	17	17	18	18
21.5	14	14	14	14	15	15	15	16	16	16	16	17	17	17	17	18	18	18
22	14	14	14	15	15	15	15	16	16	16	17	17	17	17	18	18	18	18
22.5	14	14	15	15	15	15	16	16	16	17	17	17	17	18	18	18	18	19
23	14	15	15	15	15	16	16	16	17	17	17	17	18	18	18	18	19	19
23.5	15	15	15	15	16	16	16	17	17	17	17	18	18	18	18	19	19	19
24	15	15	15	16	16	16	17	17	17	17	18	18	18	18	19	19	19	20

OF SUBSCAPULAR AND THIGH
TO PERCENTAGE OF BODY FAT

thickness (in mm)

15	15.5	16	16.5	17	17.5	18	18.5	19	19.5	20	20.5	21	21.5	22	22.5	23	23.5	24
9	10	10	10	10	11	11	11	11	12	12	12	12	13	13	13	13	14	14
10	10	10	10	11	11	11	11	12	12	12	12	13	13	13	13	13	14	14
10	10	10	11	11	11	11	12	12	12	12	13	13	13	13	14	14	14	15
10	10	11	11	11	11	12	12	12	12	13	13	13	13	14	14	14	15	15
10	11	11	11	11	12	12	12	12	13	13	13	13	14	14	14	15	15	15
11	11	11	11	12	12	12	12	13	13	13	13	14	14	14	15	15	15	15
11	11	11	12	12	12	12	13	13	13	13	14	14	14	15	15	15	15	16
11	11	12	12	12	12	13	13	13	13	14	14	14	15	15	15	15	16	16
11	12	12	12	12	13	13	13	13	14	14	14	15	15	15	15	16	16	16
12	12	12	12	13	13	13	13	14	14	14	15	15	15	15	16	16	16	16
12	12	12	13	13	13	13	14	14	14	15	15	15	15	16	16	16	16	17
12	12	13	13	13	13	14	14	14	15	15	15	15	16	16	16	16	17	17
12	13	13	13	13	14	14	14	15	15	15	15	16	16	16	16	17	17	17
13	13	13	13	14	14	14	15	15	15	15	16	16	16	16	17	17	17	17
13	13	13	14	14	14	15	15	15	15	16	16	16	16	17	17	17	17	18
13	13	14	14	14	15	15	15	15	16	16	16	16	17	17	17	17	18	18
13	14	14	14	14	15	15	15	16	16	16	16	17	17	17	17	18	18	18
14	14	14	14	15	15	15	16	16	16	16	17	17	17	17	18	18	18	18
14	14	14	15	15	15	16	16	16	16	17	17	17	17	18	18	18	19	19
14	14	15	15	15	16	16	16	16	17	17	17	17	18	18	18	19	19	19
14	15	15	15	16	16	16	17	17	17	17	18	18	18	19	19	19	19	19
15	15	15	16	16	16	16	17	17	17	17	18	18	18	19	19	19	19	20
15	15	16	16	16	16	17	17	17	17	18	18	18	19	19	19	19	20	20
15	16	16	16	16	17	17	17	17	18	18	18	19	19	19	19	20	20	20
16	16	16	16	17	17	17	17	18	18	18	19	19	19	19	20	20	20	20
16	16	16	17	17	17	17	18	18	18	19	19	19	19	20	20	20	20	21
16	16	17	17	17	17	18	18	18	19	19	19	19	20	20	20	20	21	21
16	17	17	17	17	18	18	18	19	19	19	19	20	20	20	20	21	21	21
17	17	17	17	18	18	18	19	19	19	20	20	20	20	21	21	21	21	22
17	17	17	18	18	18	18	19	19	19	20	20	20	20	21	21	21	22	22
17	17	18	18	18	18	19	19	19	20	20	20	20	21	21	21	21	22	22
17	18	18	18	18	19	19	19	20	20	20	20	21	21	21	21	22	22	22
18	18	18	18	19	19	19	20	20	20	20	21	21	21	21	22	22	22	23
18	18	18	19	19	19	20	20	20	20	21	21	21	21	22	22	22	23	23
18	18	19	19	19	20	20	20	20	21	21	21	21	22	22	22	23	23	23
18	19	19	19	20	20	20	20	21	21	21	21	22	22	22	23	23	23	23
19	19	19	20	20	20	20	21	21	21	21	22	22	22	23	23	23	23	24
19	19	20	20	20	20	21	21	21	21	22	22	22	23	23	23	23	24	24
19	20	20	20	20	21	21	21	21	22	22	22	23	23	23	23	24	24	24
20	20	20	20	21	21	21	21	22	22	22	23	23	23	23	24	24	24	25
20	20	20	21	21	21	21	22	22	22	23	23	23	23	24	24	24	25	25

TABLE 2—FEMALES: CONVERSION SKINFOLD MEASUREMENTS

Skinfold thickness at triceps (in mm)

	4	4.5	5	5.5	6	6.5	7	7.5	8	8.5	9	9.5	10	10.5	11	11.5	12	12.5
6	14	14	14	14	14	15	15	15	15	15	15	16	16	16	16	16	16	17
6.5	14	14	14	14	15	15	15	15	15	15	16	16	16	16	16	16	17	17
7	14	14	14	15	15	15	15	15	15	16	16	16	16	16	16	17	17	17
7.5	14	14	15	15	15	15	15	15	16	16	16	16	16	16	17	17	17	17
8	14	15	15	15	15	15	15	16	16	16	16	16	16	17	17	17	17	17
8.5	15	15	15	15	15	15	16	16	16	16	16	16	17	17	17	17	17	17
9	15	15	15	15	15	16	16	16	16	16	16	17	17	17	17	17	17	18
9.5	15	15	15	15	16	16	16	16	16	16	17	17	17	17	17	17	18	18
10	15	15	15	16	16	16	16	16	16	17	17	17	17	17	17	18	18	18
10.5	15	16	16	16	16	16	16	17	17	17	17	17	17	18	18	18	18	18
11	16	16	16	16	16	16	17	17	17	17	17	17	17	18	18	18	18	18
11.5	16	16	16	16	16	17	17	17	17	17	17	18	18	18	18	18	18	19
12	16	16	16	16	17	17	17	17	17	17	18	18	18	18	18	18	19	19
12.5	16	16	16	17	17	17	17	17	17	18	18	18	18	18	18	19	19	19
13	16	16	17	17	17	17	17	17	18	18	18	18	18	18	19	19	19	19
13.5	16	17	17	17	17	17	17	18	18	18	18	18	18	19	19	19	19	19
14	17	17	17	17	17	17	18	18	18	18	18	18	19	19	19	19	19	19
14.5	17	17	17	17	18	18	18	18	18	18	19	19	19	19	19	19	19	20
15	17	17	17	17	18	18	18	18	18	18	19	19	19	19	19	19	20	20
15.5	17	17	17	18	18	18	18	18	18	19	19	19	19	19	19	20	20	20
16	17	17	18	18	18	18	18	18	19	19	19	19	19	19	20	20	20	20
16.5	17	18	18	18	18	18	18	19	19	19	19	19	19	20	20	20	20	20
17	18	18	18	18	18	18	19	19	19	19	19	19	20	20	20	20	20	20
17.5	18	18	18	18	19	19	19	19	19	19	20	20	20	20	20	20	21	21
18	18	18	18	19	19	19	19	19	19	20	20	20	20	20	20	21	21	21
18.5	18	18	19	19	19	19	19	19	20	20	20	20	20	20	21	21	21	21
19	18	19	19	19	19	19	19	20	20	20	20	20	20	21	21	21	21	21
19.5	19	19	19	19	19	19	20	20	20	20	20	20	21	21	21	21	21	21
20	19	19	19	19	19	20	20	20	20	20	20	21	21	21	21	21	21	22
20.5	19	19	19	19	20	20	20	20	20	20	21	21	21	21	21	21	22	22
21	19	19	19	20	20	20	20	20	20	21	21	21	21	21	21	22	22	22
21.5	19	19	20	20	20	20	20	20	21	21	21	21	21	21	22	22	22	22
22	19	20	20	20	20	20	20	21	21	21	21	21	21	22	22	22	22	22
22.5	20	20	20	20	20	20	21	21	21	21	21	21	22	22	22	22	22	23
23	20	20	20	20	20	21	21	21	21	21	22	22	22	22	22	22	23	23
23.5	20	20	20	21	21	21	21	21	21	22	22	22	22	22	22	23	23	23
24	20	20	21	21	21	21	21	21	22	22	22	22	22	22	23	23	23	23
24.5	20	21	21	21	21	21	21	22	22	22	22	22	22	23	23	23	23	23
25	21	21	21	21	21	21	22	22	22	22	22	22	23	23	23	23	23	23
25.5	21	21	21	21	21	22	22	22	22	22	22	23	23	23	23	23	23	24
26	21	21	21	21	22	22	22	22	22	22	23	23	23	23	23	23	24	24
26.5	21	21	21	22	22	22	22	22	22	23	23	23	23	23	23	24	24	24
27	21	21	22	22	22	22	22	22	23	23	23	23	23	23	24	24	24	24

OF ILIAC CREST AND TRICEPS
TO PERCENTAGE OF BODY FAT

at iliac crest (in mm)

13	13.5	14	14.5	15	15.5	16	16.5	17	17.5	18	18.5	19	19.5	20	20.5	21	21.5	22
17	17	17	17	17	18	18	18	18	18	18	19	19	19	19	19	19	20	20
17	17	17	17	18	18	18	18	18	18	19	19	19	19	19	19	20	20	20
17	17	17	18	18	18	18	18	18	19	19	19	19	19	19	20	20	20	20
17	17	18	18	18	18	18	18	19	19	19	19	19	19	20	20	20	20	20
17	18	18	18	18	18	18	19	19	19	19	19	19	20	20	20	20	20	20
18	18	18	18	18	18	19	19	19	19	19	19	20	20	20	20	20	20	21
18	18	18	18	18	19	19	19	19	19	19	20	20	20	20	20	20	21	21
18	18	18	18	19	19	19	19	19	19	20	20	20	20	20	20	21	21	21
18	18	18	19	19	19	19	19	19	20	20	20	20	20	20	21	21	21	21
18	18	19	19	19	19	19	20	20	20	20	20	20	21	21	21	21	21	21
18	19	19	19	19	19	19	20	20	20	20	20	20	21	21	21	21	21	21
19	19	19	19	19	19	20	20	20	20	20	21	21	21	21	21	21	22	22
19	19	19	19	20	20	20	20	20	20	21	21	21	21	21	21	22	22	22
19	19	19	20	20	20	20	20	20	21	21	21	21	21	21	22	22	22	22
19	19	20	20	20	20	20	20	21	21	21	21	21	21	22	22	22	22	22
19	20	20	20	20	20	20	21	21	21	21	21	21	22	22	22	22	22	22
20	20	20	20	20	20	21	21	21	21	21	21	22	22	22	22	22	22	23
20	20	20	20	20	21	21	21	21	21	21	22	22	22	22	22	22	23	23
20	20	20	20	21	21	21	21	21	21	22	22	22	22	22	22	23	23	23
20	20	20	21	21	21	21	21	22	22	22	22	22	22	23	23	23	23	23
20	20	21	21	21	21	21	21	22	22	22	22	22	22	23	23	23	23	23
20	21	21	21	21	21	21	22	22	22	22	22	22	23	23	23	23	23	24
21	21	21	21	21	22	22	22	22	22	22	23	23	23	23	23	23	24	24
21	21	21	21	22	22	22	22	22	22	23	23	23	23	23	23	24	24	24
21	21	21	22	22	22	22	22	22	23	23	23	23	23	23	24	24	24	24
21	21	22	22	22	22	22	22	23	23	23	23	23	23	24	24	24	24	24
21	22	22	22	22	22	22	23	23	23	23	23	23	24	24	24	24	24	24
22	22	22	22	22	22	23	23	23	23	23	23	24	24	24	24	24	24	25
22	22	22	22	22	23	23	23	23	23	23	24	24	24	24	24	24	25	25
22	22	22	22	23	23	23	23	23	23	24	24	24	24	24	24	25	25	25
22	22	22	23	23	23	23	23	23	24	24	24	24	24	24	25	25	25	25
22	22	23	23	23	23	23	23	24	24	24	24	24	24	25	25	25	25	25
22	23	23	23	23	23	24	24	24	24	24	24	25	25	25	25	25	25	26
23	23	23	23	23	24	24	24	24	24	24	25	25	25	25	25	25	26	26
23	23	23	23	24	24	24	24	24	24	25	25	25	25	25	25	26	26	26
23	23	23	24	24	24	24	24	24	25	25	25	25	25	25	26	26	26	26
23	23	24	24	24	24	24	24	25	25	25	25	25	25	26	26	26	26	26
23	24	24	24	24	24	24	25	25	25	25	25	25	26	26	26	26	26	26
24	24	24	24	24	24	25	25	25	25	25	25	26	26	26	26	26	27	27
24	24	24	24	24	25	25	25	25	25	25	26	26	26	26	26	27	27	27
24	24	24	24	25	25	25	25	25	25	26	26	26	26	26	27	27	27	27
24	24	24	25	25	25	25	25	26	26	26	26	26	26	27	27	27	27	27
24	25	25	25	25	25	25	26	26	26	26	26	26	27	27	27	27	27	27

Laboratory 12

SEVEN-DAY RECORD OF CALORIC CONSUMPTION AND ENERGY EXPENDITURE

Name _____   Instructor _____

Class and section _____   Date _____

Purpose

The purpose of this laboratory session is to determine your caloric consumption and energy expenditure for a seven-day period.

Equipment Needed

None

Procedure

Maintain a record of your weight, food intake, exercise, and Calories expended for a 7-day period on pp. 232-238. Use Tables 6-6 and 6-7 for this purpose.

Results

1. Are your caloric intake and energy expenditure in balance? _____

2. Did you gain weight, lose weight, or maintain the same weight during the seven days? _____

3. Should you adjust your food intake and physical activity for good weight management? _____

4. List the more caloric-dense foods in your diet.

5. List the items that you could/would do without to reduce caloric intake.

6. Estimate the number of empty (no nutritional value) Calories consumed during the 7-day period and calculate daily average.

SUMMARY OF TOTAL CALORIC INTAKE
AND EXPENDITURE THROUGH
EXERCISE FOR SEVEN DAYS

Name _____   Body weight ____   Date _____

Instructor _____   Course & section _____

Date _____

Time	Food	Calories	Exercise & Calories Used

Date _____

Time	Food	Calories	Exercise & Calories Used

Date _____

Time	Food	Calories	Exercise & Calories Used

Date _____

Time	Food	Calories	Exercise & Calories Used

Date _____

Time	Food	Calories	Exercise & Calories Used

Date _____

Time	Food	Calories	Exercise & Calories Used

Date _____

Time	Food	Calories	Exercise & Calories Used

Laboratory 13

THE TENSE INDIVIDUAL

Name _____   Instructor _____

Class and section _____   Date _____

Purpose

The purpose of this laboratory session is to determine if you are a tense individual.

Equipment Needed

None

Procedures

1. Read each of the 25 questions listed below and check the answer that describes you most often.
2. Have a friend answer the questions to reflect how he or she perceives you.

Yes   No

_____ _____ 1. Do you often experience headaches or backaches?

_____ _____ 2. When sitting in a chair and talking to someone, do you continually move in the chair to seek a comfortable position?

_____ _____ 3. When retiring for the night, are you usually unable to fall asleep immediately?

_____ _____ 4. Do you often grind your teeth when you are confronted with an unpleasant experience?

_____ _____ 5. Do you easily become angry or frustrated when you are faced with a problem for which there is no immediate solution?

_____ _____ 6. Do you often complain of being tired?

Yes	No		
____	____	7.	Does your face often hold expressions of intense concentration?
____	____	8.	Do you often drum your fingers aimlessly or forcibly to express irritation?
____	____	9.	Does your posture appear stiff when you sit or walk?
____	____	10.	Are you unable to concentrate on one problem at a time?
____	____	11.	Are you unable to relax voluntarily?
____	____	12.	Do you often experience nervousness and uneasy feelings?
____	____	13.	Do you become upset when your plans are interrupted or must be changed?
____	____	14.	Are you highly competitive in sports, in your test grades, and in your daily responsibilities?
____	____	15.	Are you time conscious?
____	____	16.	Do you experience extreme dissatisfaction and anxiety when you fail to achieve success in your endeavors?
____	____	17.	Are you an aggressive person?
____	____	18.	Are you often too busy to allow time for physical activity?
____	____	19.	Do you plan your day's activities and often budget your time?
____	____	20.	Are you critical of yourself when you make a mistake?
____	____	21.	Do you feel "uptight" at the end of the day?
____	____	22.	Are you impatient when others are late for an appointment with you?

Yes   No

_____ _____ 23. Do you often set high goals or levels of achievement for yourself?

_____ _____ 24. Do you experience bad moods very often?

_____ _____ 25. Are you unyielding when others disagree with your beliefs or convictions?

Results

Tense people seek to release their tension in physical actions that are in no way related to the problem created by the tension. If you answered yes to many of the questions, you may need to reexamine your perception of the stressor, seek diversions to provide your worried mind with new problems that can be solved, participate in physical activity to provide a release for the tension, and participate in some form of relaxation technique.

RELAXATION TECHNIQUES

Name _____   Instructor _____

Class and section _____   Date _____

Purpose

The purpose of this laboratory session is to practice the conscious release of muscular tension (relaxation). It is a skill that is not easily performed by many individuals.

Equipment Needed

1. Mats
2. Pillows or towels

Procedures

1. Practice the Benson relaxation technique described on p. 137.
2. Have a partner or group leader guide you through the Arnheim relaxation technique described on pp. 137-139.

Results

1. Did either of the relaxation techniques help you release muscular tension? _____

2. Do you need to develop the skill to consciously relax? _____

Laboratory 15

POSTURE EVALUATION

Name _____ Instructor _____

Class and section _____ Date _____

Purpose

The purposes of this laboratory session are to evaluate your posture when standing, walking, running for distance (jogging), and lifting a heavy object, and to make you aware of postural mechanics that should be followed for each of these positions and movements.

Equipment Needed

None

Procedures

1. Wear a bathing suit if possible.
2. Work with a partner. Each evaluates the posture of the other.
3. Refer to the posture mechanics described on pp. 175-179 and use the evaluation forms to estimate your partner's posture. Score each aspect of posture as follows: no deviation, 0; slight deviation, 1; moderate deviation, 2; extreme deviation, 3.

STANDING (Refer to pp. 175-176)

1. Head and chin _____

2. Shoulders _____

3. Shoulder blades _____

4. Chest _____

5. Trunk _____

6. Abdomen _____

7. Hips _____

8. Arms _____

9. Knees _____

10. Feet _____

11. Weight _____

WALKING (Refer to p. 176)

1. Upper body _____

2. Trunk _____

3. Motion _____

4. Lead leg _____

5. Base of support _____

6. Supporting and pushing leg _____

7. Lead heel _____

8. Ankle joint of pushing leg _____

9. Weight shift _____

10. Leg muscles _____

RUNNING FOR DISTANCE (Refer to pp. 177-178)

1. Head _____

2. Back _____

3. Buttocks _____

4. Elbows _____

5. Body _____

6. Footstrike _____

SITTING (Refer to p. 178)

1. Head, neck, and shoulders _____

2. Buttocks _____

3. Feet _____

LIFTING HEAVY OBJECT (Refer to p. 178)

1. Knees and back _____

2. Feet _____

3. Lifting _____

Results

Individuals who are not trained to do so may find it difficult to evaluate posture accurately; however, this experience can provide insight into postural mechanics.

1. Are you pleased with your posture evaluation? _____

2. Should you practice better posture mechanics? _____

Laboratory 16

PREPARING A PERSONALIZED EXERCISE PRESCRIPTION

Name _____   Instructor _____

Class and section _____   Date _____

Purpose

The purpose of this laboratory session is to provide practice in preparing a personalized exercise prescription.

Equipment Needed

None

Procedure

Using the steps provided in Chapter 3 and the sample found in Appendix B, develop your own exercise prescription.

Name: _____ Age: _____ Exercise Preference: _____

Resting HR: _____ Max HR: _____

Training HR: 60% _____; 70% _____; 80% _____

CR evaluation by _____ Results: _____

Comments:

Fitness goal:

EXERCISE RECOMMENDATIONS

General:

Specific:

Exercise style & type:

Frequency:

Intensity:

Duration: